AUDIBLE BLEEDING

The Origin and

Development of the VGH

Vascular Surgery Division

YORK N. HSIANG

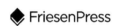 FriesenPress

Suite 300 - 990 Fort St
Victoria, BC, V8V 3K2
Canada

www.friesenpress.com

Copyright © 2021 by York N. Hsiang
First Edition — 2021

ISBN
978-1-5255-9488-5 (Hardcover)
978-1-5255-9487-8 (Paperback)
978-1-5255-9489-2 (eBook)

1. MEDICAL, SURGERY, VASCULAR

Distributed to the trade by The Ingram Book Company

Contents

Dedication

This book is dedicated to BAH—Whatever I could do, you could always make it better.

Acknowledgements

To write a book like this requires the contributions of many, and I am appreciative of all their efforts. In particular, I would like to thank my mentors, Dr. Wallace Chung and Dr. Peter Fry, who generously gave me insights into the "early days." Peter and Simon Litherland, and Hilda Hildebrand, the family members of my deceased mentors, Dr. Henry Litherland and Dr. Henry Hildebrand, provided unique stories, for which I am indebted. My colleagues and friends, Dr. David Taylor, Dr. Tony Salvian, Dr. Jerry Chen, Dr. Jason Faulds, Dr. Jon Misskey, and Dr. Joel Gagnon, all provided encouragement and many unforgettable photos. Graduates of the program, especially Drs. Gene Zierler, Albert Ting, Hamid Nasser, Mussaad Al-Salman, Musaad Al-Ghamdi, Edward Hui, Arthur Chan, and Gary Yang, provided personal stories of their travels through life and vascular surgery, which I am very thankful for. Dr. Sally Choi, a vascular surgery resident, was extremely helpful in developing videos of the surgical manoeuvres to aid the illustrator, Anzhalika Bortnik. I would like to give a special thanks to Dr. Martin McLoughlin for his keen insight into the areas where Vascular Surgery overlapped with Urology. Kathleen Murphy, president of the VGH School of Nursing Alumnae Association, provided excellent material on the history of the nursing school and books about the history of the VGH Surgery Department.

I undertook this project of documenting the origin and development of the VGH Vascular Surgery Division in December 2019 when I realized that within one year there would be a watershed moment with retirements of the senior staff. History is important. To know our place in this world and choose the correct path, we need to know where we came from, how we came to be here, and to be cognizant of the things we tried that worked or failed. This book is our history.

Introduction

Vascular Surgeons -
The Firefighters of the Operating Room

One of the most lasting images of the September 11, 2001 attack on New York City was the scene of people fighting to get out of the burning towers. Dozens were cramped in hand-to-hand combat to escape the raging inferno above. Except for the few who were going *up* the stairs. They were not terrified. Wearing their fire-retardant suits and carrying heavy hoses, the firefighters' mission was to put out the fire. Where ordinary people avoid and run from fire, there are those who, like moths, are drawn to the flame. In the operating room, when there is unexpected massive bleeding, uncontrolled—like a raging inferno—the emergency responders are the vascular surgeons.

But is there bleeding that even vascular surgeons fear? The answer is yes. My former trainee and good friend Gerrit Winkelaar told me that we should be scared of two types of bleeding: the bleeding coming from you, and *audible bleeding*. Audible bleeding is when the flow or volume of blood loss is so great you can actually hear it. Audible bleeding occurs when the aorta[1] is opened (deliberately or not), even temporarily. The gush of blood is like water from a firehose. Bleeding is also audible when the blood loss is so great, it flows out of the patient, off the OR table, and strikes the floor below. If you hear it, something has to be done. Quickly.

To be a vascular surgeon is akin to being a successful thief. It requires a high degree of training and meticulous planning. From the entry, to the taking of the goods, expecting the unanticipated, and finally escaping, without raising any alarms. But, if you get caught, you are in trouble.

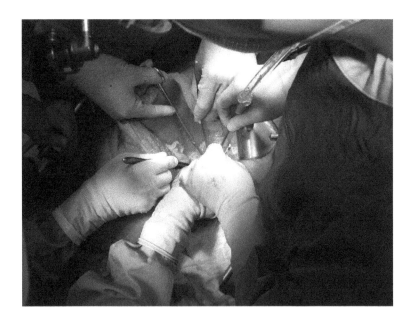

---

1   Aorta: The largest artery in the body, extending from the heart to the abdomen.

PART ONE

THE HEATHER PAVILION YEARS

(1978–1994)

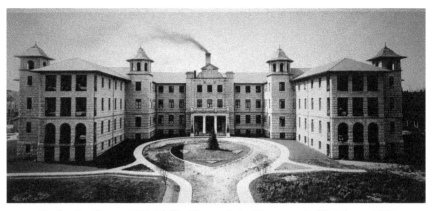

Heather Pavilion, c. 1908. Phillip Timms photo, Vancouver Public Library 5187.

When the City of Vancouver was incorporated in 1886, an initial attempt to build a small city hospital, in the area known as *Fairview*, consisted of several small tents. When these were destroyed in the Great Vancouver Fire of June 1886, the city took over the site, renamed it *Vancouver City Hospital*, and by 1899, opened a nursing school for its first class of students. In 1906, with a new board, the hospital was renamed Vancouver General Hospital (VGH) and moved to its present location from its downtown location on Beatty Street, south of Pender. With its new name, a new building was commissioned and opened, as the Heather Pavilion, to patients and medical staff in 1906, to primarily look after the wounded soldiers returning from Europe (Luxton 2006).

1

Origins

The methodical hissing of the ventilator, slurping of the suction, and periodic beeping of the alarms were nothing more than background noise that Wally tuned out. He only cared about what his eyes were showing him. He watched the expert hands of the senior surgeons before him, Dr. John Elliott and Dr. Alan (A.D.) McKenzie, rhythmically strip away all of the surrounding abdominal flesh to expose the largest artery in the body, the aorta[2].

As the senior general surgery resident, Wally had seen plenty of abdominal cases but nothing like this. Here was a patient, filleted from xiphisternum[3] to abdominal pubis[4], with his entire intestines retracted to expose the retroperitoneum[5]. And now, they were about to do something nobody in this city had ever done before. Instead of avoiding cutting into blood vessels and causing bleeding, they were going to *deliberately* cut into the aorta and replace it. The year

---

2   Aorta: Largest artery in the body, arising from the left ventricle of the heart and extending to the abdomen where it terminates into two large branches, one for each leg.
3   Xiphisternum: the lowest part of the breastbone.
4   Abdominal pubis: the lowermost region in the midline of the abdomen just above the pubic bone.
5   Retroperitoneum: The abdominal space behind the intestines, in front of the spine and back muscles.

was 1958, and these were the Vancouver pioneers who pursued the development of the specialty that operated on blood vessels: Vascular Surgery.

For decades, there had been monumental problems in the way of this new specialty. Some were fundamental questions such as, "How do you join vessels together," or "How do you replace larger vessels," and once the blood vessel had been opened, "How can you work with blood clots that form when you stop the blood flow?"

The first demonstration of how to sew blood vessels was by Alexis Carrel, a French surgeon who moved to the US to continue his work in transplantation. Carrel described the triangular suture technique for which he received the Nobel Prize in 1912 (Dente and Feliciano 2005). Despite his description of how to sew blood vessels, *modern* vascular surgery developed during wartime conflict. Prior to World War I, surgeons were performing *indirect* procedures on diseased blood vessels primarily by ligation and sympathectomy[6]. The era of *direct* reconstruction[7] began after World War II (DeBakey and Simeone 1946). Since then, a number of North American and European pioneers have developed materials and methods such as heparin for anticoagulation[8] (Couch 1989), autogenous vein grafts[9] for bypass surgery (Hess 1992), and prosthetics for large vessels[10]

6   Ligation and sympathectomy: A surgical procedure to tie off and cut the sympathetic nerves to a leg. This causes the treated side to become warmer and dryer.

7   Direct reconstruction: Traditional surgery on the blood vessel, working from outside to inside, as opposed to endovascular surgery where the surgical procedure involves working from inside of the blood vessel.

8   Heparin for anticoagulation: Heparin is a blood thinner. Anticoagulation is the process of stopping blood from clotting.

9   Autogenous vein graft: A vein removed from one part of the body and placed in another part of the body.

10   Prosthetics for large vessels: Artificial tubes designed to replace blood vessels, most commonly large vessels such as the aorta since the body does not have a similar replacement tissue.

(Smith 1993). This led to the first aortic aneurysmorrhaphy[11] in 1951 by Dubost (Dubost et al. 1951; Bergqvist 2008) and and the first carotid endarterectomy[12] in 1951 (Friedman 2014).

The founding general surgeons who were interested in advancing this new specialty of vascular surgery formed the Society for Vascular Surgery, in 1946 (Yao 2010). In the 1950s and 60s, general surgeons in many hospitals across North America formed Divisions of Vascular Surgery in their hospitals. In Canada, such divisions were forming in Montreal, Toronto, Ottawa, Winnipeg, and Edmonton.

During the late 1950's in Vancouver, Dr. John Elliott was the man with the vision for this new division. He was trained in urology and general surgery in Britain, and had served in the armed forces (Patterson 2000). Well into mid-career, Dr. Elliott had turned his attention to vascular surgery.

Of all the up-and-coming residents, Dr. Elliott chose Dr. Wallace B. Chung, or, "Wally" to his friends, to form this new division. Having demonstrated his interest in vascular surgery as a resident and after graduating from general surgery training, Wally was recruited as an assistant professor at the University of British Columbia (UBC) and as a general surgeon on staff at VGH in 1961. At that time, vascular surgical procedures consisted largely of vein strippings[13], amputations, and the occasional sympathectomy.[14]

By 1972, Wally had risen to full professor, and in 1978 was appointed by Surgery Department Head Dr. Cameron Harrison to serve as division head for both General Surgery and the new Vascular

---

11   Aortic aneurysmorrhaphy: An operation to correct an aneurysm of the aorta.
12   Carotid endarterectomy: An operation to remove plaque from the carotid artery in the neck to prevent stroke.
13   Vein strippings: Surgical procedures to remove varicose veins.
14   Sympathectomy: An operation to cut the sympathetic nerves to increase skin blood flow to the extremities.

Surgery Division. Bold surgical staff, demonstrating significant skill in the new subspecialty of vascular surgery, were recruited from the pool of general surgeons.

In 1978, there were four general surgery wards at VGH: C3 and C5 in the Heather Pavilion, and East 8 and West 8 in the Centennial Pavilion. Each of these wards had one general surgeon who also did vascular surgery. To persuade these general surgeons to participate in this new beginning, Wally assigned ward C5 in the Heather Pavilion as the new vascular surgery ward, while the other three wards would remain for general surgery cases only.

Initially, Henry Litherland, Henry Hildebrand, Anthony (Tony) Chan, and Wally Chung were to be the new vascular surgeons at VGH. A recent general surgery graduate, Peter Fry, had also shown considerable interest in cardiac and, later on, vascular surgery. However, with no further available positions at VGH, Peter applied for privileges at Lions Gate Hospital in North Vancouver.

Tragedy had struck Tony Chan and his family five years earlier. His wife, a psychiatrist, was brutally murdered by a psychotic patient in her private office close to VGH. Heartbroken, Tony informed Wally that he wished to leave VGH, now the place of indescribable pain for him and his family. Unable to convince Tony to stay, Wally approached Peter Fry about joining the newly formed group. Peter was resistant, but Wally insisted, telling him: "Try it for two years, and if you don't like it, you can leave." With this invitation, Peter joined as the fourth member of the new Vascular Surgery Division. And Tony Chan? He took Peter's position at Lions Gate Hospital where he spent the remainder of his career.

Beginnings rarely evolve uneventfully. Within several months, Litherland and Hildebrand approached Wally to express their displeasure at only being allowed to do vascular cases. They wished to maintain the old status quo by performing both general and vascular surgical cases, with their patients allowed to be kept on the vascular ward, C5. The latter had been designated as vascular-only. After a week's reflection, Wally's response was uncompromising: if vascular surgery was to move ahead as a subspecialty from general surgery then vascular surgeons would not do any elective general surgery cases.

The ultimatum was issued to Litherland and Hildebrand. They could either continue as vascular surgeons in the new subspecialty or continue to do both general and vascular cases. By choosing the latter, however, they would no longer be considered vascular surgeons and would not be allowed to admit their cases to C5. Their vacated positions would be filled. Already, a young resident named Anthony Salvian was expressing interest in the new specialty. And, a fourth would be recruited to bring the complement back up to four vascular surgeons. Furthermore, the other general surgeons would be none too happy about vascular cases being admitted to C3 and potentially blocking beds on the general surgery ward. The mini rebellion collapsed, with Litherland and Hildebrand agreeing to a practice of pure vascular surgery.

This was an example of "sticking to your guns" when you believe your cause to be just. Frequently, a leader may choose a more harmonizing compromise, wishing the problem would go away with a "Why can't we all get along?" approach. The end result was that vascular surgery at VGH flourished into its own specialty, elevating its standard over general surgery. A compromising solution would have weakened vascular surgery from the outset, and much more time would have passed before a second attempt to set it apart as a distinct specialty from general surgery.

2

GENERAL VERSUS VASCULAR SURGERY

The discipline of vascular surgery grew out of general surgery, but how are vascular surgeons different from general surgeons?

General surgeons, as their name suggests, were the original surgeons who performed surgery all over the body. Later, there was differentiation into specific systems such as orthopedics and urology. As the diseases surgeons managed could at times also be managed without surgery, medical disciplines such as gastroenterology developed alongside general surgery.

In Canada, there is no medical counterpart to vascular surgery[15] and vascular surgeons are responsible for the medical and surgical treatment of their patients. Another area of dissimilarity is in treating tumours—common for general surgeons but highly unusual for vascular surgeons. The treatment of tumours is based on the TNM[16] classification, and operations are based on these guidelines. The outcome of tumour surgery is frequently "grey" and based on health quality outcomes such as morbidity[17] and time to recurrence.

---

15   Medical counterpart: There is no doctor who treats peripheral blood vessel diseases solely with medical (drug) treatment as drug treatment is usually ineffective.
16   TNM: Acronym for tumour, node, metastasis. Used to determine the spread of cancer.
17   Morbidity: diseased state.

Vascular surgery differs from general surgery in several important areas. First, as medical treatment is largely ineffective in treating peripheral atherosclerosis[18] and aneurysms[19], surgery becomes
necessary for both palliation[20] and curative intent[21]. Second, the
indication for surgery (or no surgery) is based, not on absolute
guidelines, but on a combination of factors, including patient factors
(e.g., physiologic age, obesity, available conduit[22] etc.), risk of procedure, and anticipated surgical outcome (e.g., long-term patency[23]
or re-stenosis[24]). Unlike the outcomes[25] in general surgery, which
are frequently on a spectrum as measured by quality of life[26], the
outcomes of vascular surgery are frequently "black or white," or
dichotomous (e.g., patients either stroke or do not stroke from their
procedure). Third, rendering organs temporarily ischemic[27] while
working on their blood supply requires planning and efficient surgical movements to minimize ischemic time. This is not a requirement
in general surgery. Fourth, due to the lack of effective medical treatment for peripheral atherosclerosis and aneurysms, many high-risk
procedures are undertaken. This is reflected in vascular surgery
having the highest rate of postoperative complications of any ward

---

18   Atherosclerosis: hardening of the arteries.
19   Aneurysm: Abnormal weakening and dilation of a blood vessel, making it prone to
rupture or develop blood clots within its dilated shape.
20   Palliation: to make the patient comfortable without curing their illness.
21   Curative intent: curing illness.
22   Conduit: A bridge connecting two blood vessels. Sometimes called a bypass graft.
23   Patency: Whether a vessel is open or not. Patent = vessel that is open and not blocked.
24   Re-stenosis: Re-narrowing of a blood vessel through scarring or redevelopment
of atherosclerosis.
25   Outcomes: the results of surgery.
26   Quality of life: a measurement of how a patient is functioning, e.g., pain or physical limitations.
27   Ischemic: Devoid of blood.

in the hospital. Finally, unpredictability is common, and the vascular surgeon needs to anticipate disruptive changes in each case.

This combination of variable indications, but black or white outcomes, and unpredictability being the norm, favours those who relish challenges rather than a standard set of guidelines.

3

Town and Gown[28]

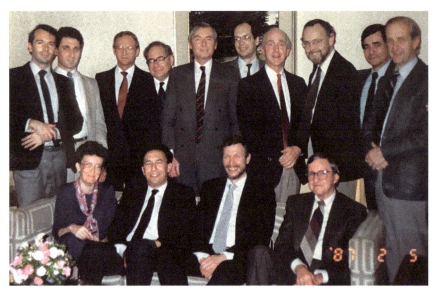

Dept. of Surgery Faculty. Back row, left to right: C. Scudamore, A. Salvian, H. Hildebrand, H. Laimon, H. Litherland, G. McGregor, A. Forward, M. G. Clay, A. Nagy, P. Fry Seated, front: J. Vestrup, J. Stoller, G. Bell, R. E. Robins. C. 1987.

The Faculty of Medicine at UBC, like many publicly funded universities, has inadequate funding to pay the salaries of its entire faculty. Initially, when both the medical school and faculty were small, faculty members were salaried, but as the number of faculty

---

28   Town and Gown: A colloquial term. *Town* refers to non-university-salaried physicians whereas *Gown* refers to university-salaried physicians.

members grew, a separate category evolved: the clinical faculty. Members of the latter were clinicians attached to one of the many affiliated teaching hospitals. Their primary role was to teach both undergraduates (medical students) and postgraduates (residents). In return, the same house staff would take primary call for the wards and the emergency room, and serve as surgical assistants if necessary. But clinical faculty were not paid a teaching stipend for many years. Eventually, they would receive an hourly stipend but only for undergraduate teaching.

In contrast, those faculty who received a salary from the university commensurate with their academic title were full-time faculty, or geographic full-time faculty (GFT)[29]. In addition to teaching, their responsibilities were either in research or education. The salaries, though, were low compared to those of full-time clinicians, and required a 20-50 percent time commitment; the remainder of their income was supplemented from clinical earnings. However, full-time faculty were members of the UBC Defined Contribution Pension Plan, and received medical, dental, and minor life insurance benefits.

Full-time faculty were periodically assessed for promotion, the rigours of which were never applied to the clinical faculty, although it had a similar promotion scheme.

These differences (earnings, focus of activity, and benefits) would become the flash points of disagreement much later, when surgeon reimbursement would change from a fee-for-service to contract model.

---

29   Geographic full time: a university-wide description of a university teacher who is paid a salary from the university.

From 1978 to 2020, there have only been four geographic full-time vascular surgeons at UBC: Drs. Wallace Chung (professor), David Taylor (associate professor), York Hsiang (professor), and Ravi Sidhu (associate professor). As these surgeons retire, their salary funding will return to the university and not to the Division of Vascular Surgery. In the future, it is highly likely that there will be no geographic full-time vascular surgeons. This may impact the future of UBC Vascular Surgery academia (see Epilogue).

Physician compensation is a flashpoint if there is significant disparity between individuals doing very similar things. Should an hour of teaching or research be paid the same as an hour in the clinic or the operating room? If you believe it should, then creating a contract to pay members who do diverse but equal things makes sense. If not, then it's nearly impossible to create a contract applicable to vastly different sources of earnings. (See chapter entitled "What is a Surgeon's Time Worth?")

4
—

Beginning of a New Subspecialty

The new subspecialty of vascular surgery required a new paradigm for training. Initially, it required a fellowship. Administered through the Royal College of Physicians and Surgeons of Canada, this program required that graduates of either general or cardiothoracic surgery to apply for an additional year of training in vascular surgery at an approved educational site. During this time, fellowship trainees would focus completely on the intellectual and technical development required to become a competent vascular surgeon. From the 1960s to 1990s, surgical treatment of large vessel problems was done directly, or using *open* surgical techniques[30]. The candidates would then have to pass an oral examination at the completion of the year's training to receive a diploma for this new designation: Special Competence in Vascular Surgery.

The first group of Canadian surgeons took this new exam in 1983. Since none of the vascular surgeons could be "grandfathered," for the first year of the exam, Peter Fry was the only candidate from BC and Wally Chung served as an examiner. On the flight to the exam centre in Ottawa, Peter read Wally's classic paper on carotid body

---

30   Open surgical techniques: traditional surgery

tumours (Chung 1979). As luck would have it, Peter's exam question was about carotid body tumours. Having thoroughly impressed the examiners, Peter was considered "a genius" by the examining committee. Inside, Wally must have been beaming.

The following year, the roles were reversed, with Wally Chung being the candidate and Peter Fry, the chief examiner. Knowing there would be a focus on medical treatments on the exam, Peter repeatedly placed articles on medical treatments for vascular disease on Wally's desk. Unconvinced that the exam would focus on medical treatments, Wally largely ignored those articles. However, as predicted by Peter, the exam did contain a number of questions on medical treatments. So, when a question was asked of Wally about calcium channel blockers,[31] everybody heard Wally exclaim, "God damn you, Fry!"

Over the next twenty-two years, the vascular fellowship became a two-year fellowship, and the exam was expanded into written and oral components. But nothing ever matched the shenanigans of the first two years of the fellowship exam.

---

31   Calcium channel blocker: A type of medication that works on the calcium channels in the heart to slow down the heart and relax the constriction on blood vessels.

5

THE UBC VASCULAR SURGERY
FELLOWSHIP PROGRAM

After minting the experienced vascular surgeons, a vascular fellow-ship program was started at UBC in 1985. It initially consisted of twelve months of pure clinical vascular surgery after five years of general surgery. At the time, the fifth year of general surgery was an elective year with final year residents being allowed to continue with general surgery rotations or pursue research, other interests, or both. To be a vascular fellow required a candidate to have satis-factorily completed a general surgery residency. But, as the general surgery exam was not until the fall and the vascular fellowship started in July of the same year, fellows accepted into the vascular surgery fellowship program were allowed to start their clinical fel-lowship year during the final year of general surgery training and write the general surgery examination three to four months later. That proved to be a problem for two fellows who were not able to pass their general surgery exams and had to be terminated from the vascular surgery fellowship.

Training was initially divided between the Vancouver teaching hospitals: VGH, UBC Hospital (UBCH), and St. Paul's Hospital (SPH). From 2014 onwards, other training sites throughout B.C., such as in Victoria, Kelowna, Richmond, and the Royal Columbian Hospital in New Westminster, have also started to have regular vascular surgery rotations.

VGH was always the largest site, with its complement of four surgeons: Henry Litherland, Henry Hildebrand, Peter Fry, and Anthony (Tony) Salvian. UBCH initially consisted of Wally Chung and Peter Fry, but later Lynn Doyle and I were added to its teaching staff. Following the merger of UBCH and VGH, the VGH surgical staff expanded to six after the retirements of Wally Chung and Lynn Doyle.

At St. Paul's, both the hospital and vascular surgery service were smaller than those of VGH, but being the downtown trauma hospital, it was very busy and had a burgeoning dialysis centre. Joseph (Joe) Sladen and Thomas (Tom) Maxwell were the founding surgeons. Years later, Jock Reid, Shaun MacDonald and Ravi Sidhu would join as staff surgeons.

Peter Fry was the first program director and would become the chief examiner for the Royal College of Physicians and Surgeons' Special Competency Examination in Vascular Surgery. In later years, a number of other UBC surgeons would assume the mantle of chief examiner, including David Taylor, Jerry Chen, and Joel Gagnon.

Lynn Doyle was selected to be the first fellow of the program. She would also become the first female vascular surgeon in Canada. Upon graduation, Lynn spent six months at Cedars Sinai Hospital in Los Angeles and worked with the eccentric Warren Grundfest.

Upon returning to Vancouver, she was given a staff position in the new vascular surgery unit at UBCH, headed by Wally Chung.

The following year saw the largest cohort of fellows—three: David Taylor, John (Jock) Reid, and Annette Holmvang. After graduating, Dave spent a year with Dr. Eugene Strandness in Seattle, and Jock did a year of trauma surgery at Parkland Hospital, Dallas. Annette started her practice in Richmond, BC where she spent her entire career. Upon completion of their additional fellowships, David was recruited to VGH and Jock to SPH.

I was the fellow in the 1987-88 year. Following that, I completed a master's in health care and epidemiology at UBC before spending an extra six months of research training under the tutelage of Dr. Rodney White at Harbor-UCLA. Harbor was a hotbed for endovascular[32] innovations, including the hot tip argon beam laser, intravascular[33] ultrasound, and laser fusion of blood vessels. I was recruited in 1989 to replace Wally Chung, who graciously stepped aside and gave me his hospital resources.

In the early 1990s, Dr. Tony Salvian was approached by a grateful patient, William Rogers. He was an engineer who believed in the importance of research, and generously donated a funded research position in addition to the one-year vascular surgery fellowship. This became the Robert C. and Patricia F. Rogers Fellowship (named after his parents), and all fellows would undergo an initial year of research followed by a year of clinical vascular surgery. The first Rogers fellow was Dr. Jerry Chen. With the funded research position, this period was the zenith of research productivity for the Division.

---

32 Endovascular: a new method of vascular surgery, operating from within the blood vessel.
33 Intravascular: within the blood vessel.

Key studies from the Rogers Fellowship years focused clinically on diverse vascular issues such as the diagnostic criteria for ultrasound to detect carotid artery stenosis[34] (Chen et al. 1998), clinical predictors of death in patients with ruptured abdominal aortic aneurysm (AAA) (Chen et al. 1996), as well as the first case report on multiple vascular occlusions[35] due to cocaine (Chen et al. 1996). Our non-clinical research was focused on a novel way to treat atherosclerosis—using photodynamic therapy[36] (Hsiang et al. 1995), and the role of the local peptide hormone, somatostatin, in vascular disease[37] (Curtis et al. 2000).

In 2001, the Royal College mandated that the vascular fellowship be a two-year clinical fellowship. The expansion was necessary because of the need to incorporate endovascular training. The postgraduate office agreed, and provided the funds to increase the fellowship to two years. With the change, however, the one-year Rogers research fellowship year was eliminated. Thus ended the enrichment year of research for the fellows and a significant amount of the division's academic output.

Giving credit wherever credit is due may not be enough. To give credit its proper due, and to establish provenance, documentation is fundamental.

---

34   Carotid artery stenosis: a narrowing of the carotid artery (in the neck).

35   Occlusions: blockages.

36   Photodynamic therapy: a treatment using a light-sensitive drug and light of a specific wavelength.

37   Somatostatin (role in vascular disease): somatostatin, an inhibitory hormone, blocks the growth of blood vessels.

6

Carotid Endarterectomy:

The Index Procedure for Vascular Surgery

All surgical specialties have an index procedure, usually the most technically challenging, often reserved as the last procedure for a trainee surgeon to undertake completely; the results used for comparison or bragging rights. For vascular surgery, that procedure is carotid endarterectomy.

An extremely technically demanding procedure, it requires precision and delicate handling of tissues. The careful dissection is often described as "dissecting the artery away from the patient" in order to minimize disturbance to the carotid artery. The consequences of failing to do a perfect procedure may lead to a devastating stroke. Even technically perfect procedures can end up with a stroked patient, emphasizing the unpredictable nature of vascular surgery.

The first carotid reconstruction[38] for stroke was described by Carrea, Molins, and Murphy in 1951. However, the first carotid

---

38   Carotid reconstruction: when the carotid artery narrows due to atherosclerotic plaque, the narrowing as well platelet adherence on the plaque can cause stroke if a portion of the plaque breaks off, or if the narrowing restricts blood flow to the brain. Reconstructing the carotid artery requires removing the plaque and leaving a smooth inner surface on the carotid artery.

endarterectomy was reportedly done by Dr. Hugh Eastcott in the United Kingdom in 1954, and by Dr. Michael DeBakey in the United States in 1953 (Thompson 1997). In Vancouver, with the new field of vascular surgery gaining momentum under John Elliott, Wally Chung was chosen to visit the famous Dr. DeBakey in 1958 to observe how this new procedure should be performed. After his return, in 1959, Wally did the first endarterectomy in Vancouver. By 1967, he had satisfactorily completed dozens of these procedures and reported his series of 78 carotid endarterectomies in 60 patients (Chung 1967).

As the number of endarterectomies increased, other surgeons from cardiac to neurosurgery tried to emulate Wally's outstanding results on their own patients. Faced with several early strokes and realizing how quickly bad news spread throughout the operating room, both cardiac and neurosurgery slowly gave up the practice of carotid endarterectomy.

Based on the difference in surgical results, carotid endarterectomy at VGH to this day is almost exclusively done by the vascular surgeons. In 2010, Tony Salvian reviewed our group's experience from 2006 to 2010. There were 501 carotid endarterectomies performed during this period with an overall mortality of 0.02% and stroke rate of 0.8% (unpublished data).[39] Thus, the tradition of excellence has been maintained many years after Wally Chung introduced carotid endarterectomy to Vancouver.

How do you stay alive in this business? You have to be good and stay good.

---

39   Published data show that high quality centres should have a combined stroke and death rate of less than 2%.

7

The Loss of Transplantation

The story of the development of transplantation is a fascinating one, arising from observations from investigators interested in infectious disease, cancer, normal immunity, and genetics (Brent 1997).

Surgeons also played a prominent role in transplantation history. The earliest surgeon to dabble in transplantation was John Hunter, a Scottish anatomist and surgeon, who wished to determine if the male organ would grow in females by transplanting the cock testes into the abdomen of both the native cock and the hen. These and other Hunterian experiments are kept in the museum named after him in the Royal College of Surgeons of England in London (Brent 1997).

Famous (and Nobel Prize-winning) for developing the triangular suture technique for vascular anastomosis[40], Alexis Carrel was a pioneering French surgeon who moved to New York to work at the Rockefeller Institute. Instead of studying skin transplantation, which was the main focus at that time, Carrel was interested in kidney transplants. He successfully transplanted kidney allografts in dogs and cats, which most typically lasted no more than a few weeks (Brent 1997).

---

40   Vascular anastomosis: the joining of blood vessels by sewing them together.

Progress in transplantation was rapid over the next five decades, with the development of anti-rejection drugs. The first successful human kidney transplant was performed in the United States in 1954 (Harvard Gazette 2011). Worldwide, all of the prominent transplant surgeons were general surgeons with a specific interest in vascular surgery. From the 1960s to 1980s, vascular surgeons were being called on to do transplants, and this new surgical technique blossomed with the return of Dr. Martin (Marty) McLoughlin to Vancouver.

Marty was born in Vancouver and attended the UBC Medical School. As an intern he showed great promise for a surgical career, and chose urology. By the late 1960s, kidney transplantation had been performed for over ten years, although few centres were specialized to do this. In 1968, as an intern, Marty had the good fortune to work with Dr. Tom Starzl, a pioneer surgeon scientist at the University of Colorado, before completing his urology residency and continuing as faculty at the Johns Hopkins University in Baltimore.

Marty was recruited back to VGH and UBC as a full professor of surgery in 1977. At the time, kidney transplantation was done as a group effort by the vascular surgeons and urologists. The vascular surgeon's role was re-attaching the renal artery and vein to the recipient's iliac artery and vein, and the urologist's role was procuring the organ and attaching the ureter to the bladder. Marty was the first surgeon in Vancouver who could do both the vascular and urological parts of the procedure. In addition, through his work with Starzl, he was a member of the American Transplant Society.

These qualities endeared him to the transplant nephrologists[41], Drs. John Price and Ted Reeves, who preferentially referred transplant cases to him. Marty also trained the urologists, including Dr. Jamie Wright, to do kidney transplants. Price wanted a more academic focus in the approach to kidney transplantation and decreed that all physicians, both internists and surgeons, needed to have a focused interest in this area, and preferably belong to the American Transplant Society (ATS). On the Medicine side, Dr. Paul Keown was recruited, and Ted Reeves was let go as transplant director. Urologists such as Dr. Lorne Sullivan, who did not belong to the ATS, were told they should no longer do kidney transplants.

For the vascular surgeons, the question was whether any of them would consider additional training to become a member of the ATS or give up their technical role in the procedure. None of the surgeons were willing to take on the challenge of additional training; thus, the Vascular Surgery Division stopped their involvement in organ transplantation. Within a few years, Dr. Chris Shackleton, a nephrologist-turned-surgeon, and trained by the vascular surgeons, would become part of the transplant faculty.

To this day, the vascular surgeons are not involved in transplantation, whether it is organ procurement or transplanting the organ. However, if there is a surgical emergency due to either bleeding or thrombosis, the vascular surgeons are frequently consulted to correct the problem.

Change is inevitable. Either adapt or get out of the way. This is a recurring theme and will be revisited under "Bringing Endovascular to VGH."

---

41   Transplant nephrologists: kidney specialists with specialized interests in kidney transplantation.

8

Ultrasound -
The First Skirmish with Radiology

As the endovascular fellow at the Cleveland Clinic (see "Bringing Endovascular to VGH"), I was surrounded by many international fellows, including those from cardiac surgery. Despite knowing how to sew arteries and veins, the approach to the two specialties could not be more different.

The practice of vascular surgery is honed by ultrasound. It is used for almost all cases. From simple ankle-brachial indices[42], to venous reflux and vein mapping in preparation for arterial surgery, it provides the physiologic and anatomic information decisions are based on.

The other way of looking at ultrasound is that vascular surgery treats abnormal anatomy *and* physiology that causes symptoms, rather than simply fixing structural problems. Without adequate grounding in the understanding of ultrasound and how it guides our decision-making process, all of the cardiac surgery fellows I met struggled during the endovascular fellowship.

---

42   Ankle-brachial indices: a ratio comparison of blood pressures between the ankle and the upper arm.

The history of the application of ultrasound to medicine, and particularly vascular surgery, started in the 1960s through developments in Japan and the United States. Doppler ultrasound and waveform analysis, followed by duplex ultrasound and colour Doppler scanning have made ultrasound the preferred non-invasive imaging modality (Siegel 1998).

Peter Fry recognized the importance of ultrasound in the late 1970s, especially the use of an ultrasound arteriograph[43] to potentially replace diagnostic angiography[44]. He encouraged a general surgery resident originally from the US, Gene Zierler, to visit Dr. Eugene Strandness, the leading authority on the use of ultrasound in vascular surgery, at the University of Washington. For over twenty years, Dr. Strandness had been a pioneer in ultrasound research from its early development to everyday use in clinical care. Gene's eyes were opened after visiting him; after graduating from general surgery, Gene returned to Seattle to continue working with Dr. Strandness (see Gene's story under "Graduates of the Vascular Surgery Program").

Ultrasound machines have never been cheap. Instead of waiting for traditional routes of requesting new capital equipment, Peter Fry, while at UBCH in 1980, successfully fundraised almost $250,000 for a new machine (see "Fundraising and Awards"). Through a process of matched funding, two ultrasound machines were purchased: one for UBCH and the other for the veteran's hospital, Shaughnessy Hospital. The latter institution had served veterans as well as civilians from both World Wars since 1917. Despite its value in treating

---

43 Ultrasound arteriograph: an intriguing concept that never developed into routine clinical use.

44 Diagnostic angiography: an invasive procedure that requires injecting X-ray dye into a blood vessel. It remains one of the standard methods of diagnosing vascular disease.

an ever-increasing number of civilians, Shaughnessy Hospital was closed in 1993. Its functions and assets were divided amongst the other Vancouver hospitals.

When he was the vascular fellow, David Taylor also developed a keen interest in ultrasound. He planned to learn more about the technology by spending an additional year of training under Dr. Strandness and bring this knowledge back to VGH. David's wish to add ultrasound to the Vascular Lab at VGH complicated our relationship with radiology. Despite obtaining a grant from BC Tel to purchase a state-of-the-art Accuson ultrasound machine, training to operate the machine, and interpret its images, this move was unacceptable to the radiologists.

Traditionally, ultrasound has been used by radiologists as an important diagnostic imaging modality. David wanted to place a new ultrasound machine in the Vascular Lab, where previously only non-imaging studies such as pressure waveform measurements[45] had been done. The radiologists saw this as an attempt to subvert their specialty of imaging. Led by Radiology Department Head Joaquin Burhenne, and supported by radiologists Peter Cooperberg and Jean Buckley, they argued that Dave should not be allowed to operate an ultrasound purely for vascular surgery because as a single physician he would not be able to adequately supervise technicians if there was nobody else on site to address issues. Also, they argued, there were no professional billing codes for ultrasound imaging that non-radiologists such as vascular surgeons could use.

Surgery Department Head A. D. (Herb) Forward and Vascular Surgery Division Head Henry Litherland were supportive of Dave's

---

45   Pressure waveform measurements: A non-invasive method of analysing blood flow with each heartbeat. If the blood pressure within the vessel is normal, a characteristic waveform is recognized. If the blood pressure is low, the waveform will be low, or *dampened.*

position. However, as there were no other vascular surgeons who had similar expertise in ultrasound, the requirement of continuous on-site supervision could not be addressed, and the surgeons had to concede that this was not possible. This stopped the expansion of vascular labs in BC, unlike elsewhere in Canada and the US.

For all those wishing to expand, remember, we are all connected. What appears to be a gain for you may be a loss for somebody else. As vascular surgeons, we thought this would be an advance for our patients and practices. The radiologists, however, perceived this as an intrusion into their sphere of practice. To have been more successful, a dialogue could have been established between Vascular Surgery and Radiology to develop mutually beneficial goals for this new technology.

9
—

Who Killed Rotating Internship?

If you ask any physician who graduated before 1990 which was the best year of their medical career, they will tell you without hesitation it was the year of rotating internship. Why? Well, there are a number of reasons. First, after slogging through medical school, being an intern meant you were free to stop reading every night. In fact, all those "facts" disappeared as fast as receding light. In its place, new "facts" based on rational thought, and later, experience, would take over. To simply survive internship, certain activities had to be prioritized—like eating whenever you could, using the bathroom whenever you saw it, or sleeping whenever possible.

Those days were long and busy, but not draconian. Instead, there was freedom in being unleashed to write orders, prescriptions, and personal recommendations because now *your* opinion mattered. Patients, nurses, even the floor cleaners called you *Doctor*. Oh, how that silly six-letter word became your prized possession! Your new status was announced to the world by a full-length white coat instead of those half-length bum-freezers. And to make sure everybody within earshot was aware of your importance, you were issued

. . . . a beeper! Perhaps most significant of all, you were actually paid (albeit not much) to do the tasks of your chosen career.

By the end of the internship year, interns would write the licensing exam. A pass would entitle them to become "real" doctors, opening new doors to start a family practice, work as a locum in various parts of the country and the world, or choose a residency.

And that was also the problem, since the College of Family Physicians of Canada had a two year post graduate certificate program and considered their graduates to be specialists in family practice. Given the choice of either one or two years to become a family physician, most chose the former. After a presumed long period of discussion with the Royal College of Physicians and Surgeons of Canada, the College of Family Physicians' recommendation that all new family physicians would require a certificate in family practice was accepted, and the one-year internship was abolished.

From 1994 onwards, this action had a dramatic deleterious downstream effect. Instead of residency being an option for those who did not want to practice family medicine, getting into a residency program now became a requirement of every medical student well before graduation. Medical student electives thus became much more focused on getting students into their residency of choice rather than helping them develop a broader understanding of medicine (Gupta, Palmer, and Cheeseman 2003).

Focusing on a career path was not the only problem for medical students. Many years earlier, all medical schools had abolished letter or numeric grades. Without grades, how can medical students distinguish themselves? The only ways are by the number of rotations in a specific specialty (to demonstrate "serious interest"), letters of reference, and the interview for residency.

Following the interviews, medical students list their preferred choices of residency programs and each residency program similarly lists its preferred choices of applicants. Through a computerized matching system, students are matched to a residency program. However, not all students are matched and around 10 percent of all graduating medical students in Canada go unmatched.

This enormous challenge has led to considerable stress for medical students, since being unmatched means that the new graduate is effectively unemployed—being labelled a doctor but not being able to practice. This has led unmatched newly minted physicians to scramble to find something relevant to do until the next match cycle the following year. Some unmatched graduates may choose to pursue a master's program if they are able to register in time. Others may seek medical research opportunities. And some may simply volunteer to do anything medical. But, for all of them there is constant fear, anxiety, and depression if they do not get matched the following year. This has even led to the occasional suicide of unfortunate unmatched new physicians who are continually denied a residency position (Glauser 2018).

What was once the highlight of one's medical career has become the horror of not knowing—not knowing if you will get into a residency, not knowing if you chose the right residency, and not knowing what you don't know.

We have all heard about creatures who eat their young. In Medicine, this is the most glaring example. How could a group of well-informed physicians knowingly eliminate the best year of a physician's life? Nobody ever did a study to determine if family physicians who completed only one post graduate year (internship) were any less knowledgeable, competent, or qualified than their counterparts who spent two post graduate years. Even worse is recognizing an error but failing to acknowledge or correct it. To this day, physicians who recognize this blight have remained silent, to the anguish of their young.

PART TWO

UNIVERSITY HOSPITAL YEARS

(1980–2003)

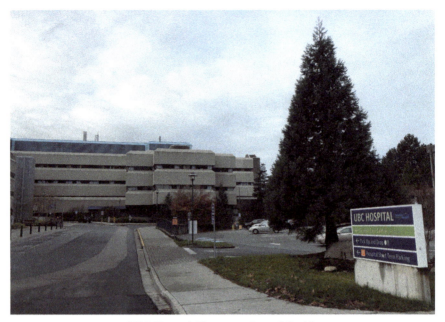

UBC Hospital. Vancouver Coastal Health.

The concept of a university hospital on the UBC campus, a stone's throw from the basic science Departments, was the brainchild of Frank Wesbrook. Originally designed in 1968, University Hospital was finally completed in 1980 with 300 beds. Being out on the peninsula where UBC sits on its Endowment Land, it had a "country club" atmosphere quite distinct from the hustle and bustle of the other major adult hospitals, VGH and St. Paul's. Not being a trauma centre nor having a dialysis program will do that to any hospital. Vascular surgery was the flagship surgical service and Wally Chung was the first department head of Surgery as well as the division head of Vascular Surgery.

Its new vascular surgery faculty with Wally, Peter Fry, Lynn Doyle, and later, me (I replaced Wally Chung), were all recently trained and had a spirit of adventure, having completed fellowships in the

US. With fewer restrictions and personalities to deal with, and later joined by equally young and eager faculty such as Lindsay Machan and Mike Martin in Radiology, the hospital became a hotbed of activity. Vascular surgery was already slowly changing from standard open procedures to endovascular procedures including angioplasty and stents, after the descriptions by Dotter and Palmaz (Friedman 1989, UC Davis Health 2010). Other new devices such as angioscopes, atherectomy catheters, intravascular ultrasound, and lasers were being added to the armamentarium of vascular surgeons. Vascular surgery in the late 1980s and early 1990s was a heady mix of excitement from new, largely untested devices and cautionary disapproval from elder surgeons.

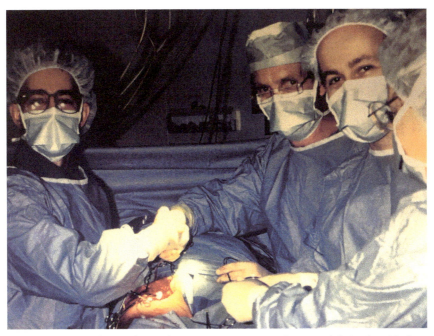

Another joint Radiology and Vascular Surgery success at UBCH. From left, Lindsay Machan, Peter Fry, David Ratliff. c. 1989.

The philosophy of the vascular surgeons of University Hospital, or UBCH, was definitely in the new and exciting endovascular camp. In 1989, UBCH was the site of the inaugural Vancouver Symposium

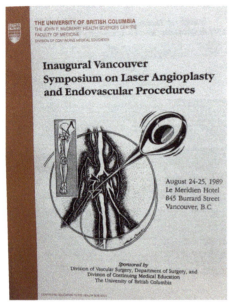

THE UNIVERSITY OF BRITISH COLUMBIA
THE JOHN P. McCREARY HEALTH SCIENCES CENTRE
FACULTY OF MEDICINE
DIVISION OF CONTINUING MEDICAL EDUCATION

Inaugural Vancouver Symposium on Laser Angioplasty and Endovascular Procedures

August 24-25, 1989
Le Meridien Hotel
845 Burrard Street
Vancouver, B.C.

Sponsored by
Division of Vascular Surgery, Department of Surgery, and
Division of Continuing Medical Education
The University of British Columbia

on Laser Angioplasty and Endovascular Procedures.

For the meeting, renowned international speakers including Drs. Rodney White, Edward Diethrich, and Geoff White were invited. Canada's first laser (argon beam) angioplasty[46] case was also performed at UBCH in 1989 and the first endovascular stent[47] graft (EVAR)[48] implanted in 1997.

As predicted, based on the hospital's proximity to the main UBC campus, research collaborations developed between Physiology, Anatomy, Pharmacology, Pathology, and Mechanical Engineering. Initially, the studies were focused on pathologic changes in atherosclerosis (Hsiang et al. 1994) and novel endovascular treatments (Hsiang et al. 1995) but later collaborations focused on the hemodynamic changes[49] seen in vascular diseases and their treatments (Schajer et al. 1996).

---

46   Angioplasty: widening of a blood vessel; can be done either by traditional surgery or internally using a balloon catheter.
47   Stent: a metal scaffold used to prop open the vessel wall.
48   Endovascular stent graft (EVAR): a stent covered by fabric inserted to line the inside of the blood vessel.
49   Hemodynamic changes: fluid mechanical forces such as blood pressure and flow.

These collaborations had a profound effect, especially on Mechanical Engineering colleagues Sheldon Green and Gary Schajer, whose main research focus was in wood and steel experiments. There, the variances were extremely small. Human biology, in contrast, had huge variations, and the concept of maintenance of a round or oval shape in the presence of no luminal blood was fascinating to every engineer who touched a collapsed empty vein compared with a contracted but still non-

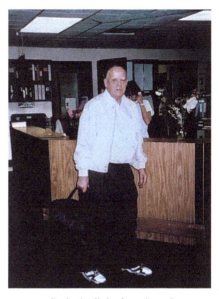

"What's all the fuss about?"
Mr. E. H., the first EVAR patient in Canada, going home the day after his procedure. c. 1997.

collapsed artery. These collaborations would prove to be very useful, with the development of the Vascular Engineering Research Group (VERG) many years later.

The good times at UBCH could not last however, because of city-wide pressures to close Shaughnessy Hospital in 1993, with the absorption of its patients into the remaining adult hospitals, and movement of personnel across the city through attrition. In the same year, UBCH was merged with VGH to form the Vancouver Hospital and Health Sciences Centre (VHHSC). Initially, not too much changed, but slowly the acquisition of the smaller UBCH led to its transformation from a medium-sized acute care hospital to a smaller hospital primarily for outpatient surgery and medical clinics, an emergency room mainly for campus and Point Grey residents, and some medical wards. Its many vacated physician and clinic office spaces were re-developed for brain and cardiology research.

By 1994, Henry Litherland retired, and I was recruited to VGH. UBCH, now reduced to only two vascular surgeons, would no longer be a leader in vascular surgery research. With the amalgamation reducing UBCH to a shell of its former self, Vascular Surgery was officially closed, with Peter Fry and Lynn Doyle moving to VGH in 2003.

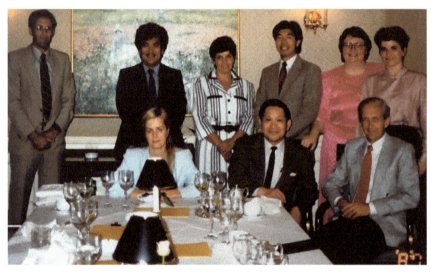

UBCH Staff Dinner. Back, Left to Right: Cedric Carter (Hematology), John Yu (DVL), Doris Wright (DVL), York Hsiang (Fellow), Mary Lou Christensen (Head Nurse), unknown female. Front, Left to Right: Lynn Doyle, Wally Chung, Peter Fry. c. 1987.

PART THREE

THE CENTENNIAL PAVILION YEARS

(1994–2003)

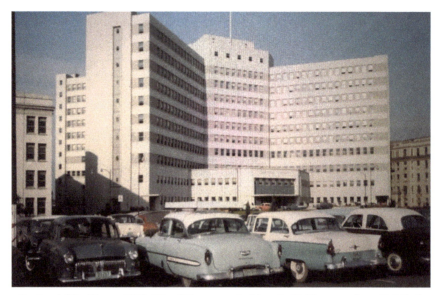

Centennial Pavilion, c. 1959. City of Vancouver Archives. Leslie Sheraton photo. Ref. Code AM1517-S1-: 2008-022.073

In 1959, a new pavilion was designed at VGH. Named *Centennial*, to commemorate British Columbia's centennial as a British Crown Colony (1858), it had four wings radiating in four directions, with a central core. Initially, the Centennial operating rooms were used by all surgeons, including the vascular surgeons. By 1994, vascular surgery moved from ward C5 in Heather Pavilion to West 8, in Centennial Pavilion. This iconic building was renamed *Blackmore Pavilion* in 2017, in honour of Leon Judah Blackmore.

The next nine years, until vascular surgery moved into the Jim Pattison Tower in 2003, were highlighted by key events; some were subtle, while others loudly declared their arrival.

10

WHEN MRSA CAME TO TOWN

The methicillin-resistant *Staphylococcus aureus*, or MRSA, came quietly but hit VGH like a maelstrom in 1997. The first patient was a dialysis patient who had recently travelled back from the Punjab. It was alleged that antibiotic prescription practices were abusive in India, with patients going to pharmacies requesting antibiotics. If one antibiotic did not work, the patient returned in a few days and requested a new antibiotic. It was alleged that this antibiotic abuse promoted resistance.

The same patient ended up on the Vascular Surgery service, as they commonly do, with either a vascular access issue or an ischemic problem, usually involving the feet. From there, the bacteria spread to the operating room, dialysis unit, ICU, and throughout the hospital.

We first noticed that something was amiss when typical wound infections would not heal as expected. Superficial wound infections became deep wound infections, and if they were over bypass grafts, either prosthetic or autogenous, the results were uniformly disastrous. Grafts were blowing out on the ward, necessitating urgent take-backs to the OR for revision or ligation.

Initial attempts at stopping the infection included isolation, hand hygiene, and use of personnel protective equipment (PPE) for the medical and nursing staff. Hand hygiene became an essential requirement before and after visiting the patient. New hand basins had to be added to the ward, including the new step-down unit, a unit created for primarily abdominal aortic aneurysm (AAA) and carotid patients. Hand disinfectants were also promoted for those times when soap and water was not available. Although Infection Control had the information from hand imprints, the actual results of who had dirty hands even after supposed hand washing was never disclosed.

How effective were the isolation attempts? It was hard to know since the number of cases was continually increasing. Many of the foreign-trained fellows, especially those from Hong Kong where MRSA was endemic, laughed at our fussing with isolation, gowning, and gloving for patients. Apparently, all their staff were issued portable hand sanitizers to use, and when empty, they were replenished. In Vancouver, portable hand sanitizers would become available only at a later stage.

Every unit of the hospital was involved, and we learned many of their practices. The plastic surgeons coined the term, "melting graft syndrome" when their split-thickness skin grafts disintegrated (hence, the term *melting graft*) with MRSA infection. From Dr. Doug Courtemanche and the plastic surgeons, we learned the virtue of adequate soft tissue coverage over our vein and prosthetic grafts. As a result, the sartorius myoplasty[50] became one of the early tissue transfer procedures that the vascular surgeons learned, and would pass on to the residents.

---

50   Sartorius myoplasty: a surgical repair using the sartorius muscle of the leg.

From Dr. Bas Masri and the orthopedic surgeons, we learned the value of sterilizing the wound bed following debridement[51] and irrigation, the use of antibiotic beads for a very high local concentration of antimicrobials, and the need to take back patients frequently for further debridement.

New procedures such as re-routing grafts through non-infected fields were now frequently discussed. For limb bypasses, whether to use an *in situ* or reversed vein technique[52] became much more relevant in a patient whose saphenous vein was very superficial. By that time, we had all seen the ravages of a superficial wound infection that arose from an infected hematoma[53] or seroma[54], only to become a deep wound infection that surrounded the bypass graft.

All of these were examples of changing behaviour to adapt to a changing situation. A good crisis will do that to you. Two key behavioural changes, one successful and the other not so much, developed in response to the repeated episodes of graft rupture and hemorrhage. The first was changing the standard vertical groin incision recommended by every vascular surgery textbook, to gain exposure of the underlying femoral vessels[55]. A vertical incision in the groin was simple ("There is nothing important superficial to the femoral artery and vein,"—Henry D. Hildebrand), provided excellent exposure, and was easy to close. A vertical incision, especially in an obese

---

51   Debridement: surgical treatment to remove dead tissue.

52   *In situ* or reversed vein technique: When using the great saphenous vein in the leg to bypass a blockage in the same leg, the saphenous vein can either be removed and turned around ("reversed") so that the vein valves are now in the direction of flow; or can be left in place ("in situ"), but an additional instrument has to be inserted to cut the vein valves so they do not obstruct flow.

53   Hematoma: a collection of blood outside of the blood vessel into the surrounding tissue; a bruise.

54   Seroma: a collection of inflammatory fluid in the soft tissue.

55   Femoral vessels: the femoral artery and vein in the groin.

patient with a pannus[56] that hangs over the inguinal fold, was neither easy to open nor close up afterwards—especially given that some folds had yeast growing underneath them. For those patients, having a groin wound infection was expected.

Enter the transverse groin incision along Langer's lines[57]. In patients with a large pannus, the incision was now on the anterior surface of the pannus which meant that the incision could be inspected without undue manipulation and could also be exposed to air after a few post-op days. This incision, however, took longer, was deeper, was more technically challenging, and gave limited visibility to anything distal[58] to the femoral bifurcation[59]. But it was better for the patient. During the height of the early days with MRSA, our femoral crossover bypass[60] infection rates were at least 10 percent. When utilizing a transverse incision for a femoral crossover bypass, even in a very slim patient with minimal subcutaneous fat, I have not seen a deep infection requiring graft excision in my patients.

The other behavioural change I wanted the residents to make was in the timing of when a dressing was removed to examine the wound. The best dressing is the one done in the operating room, since it is applied by the surgeon in the most sterile environment. After that, all dressing changes pale in comparison. So, whenever a dressing is removed on the ward post-op, it is an invitation for

---

56   Pannus: an apron of fatty tissue.
57   Langer's lines: Typological lines of skin tension that parallel the orientation of collagen fibres in the skin and the underlying muscle.
58   Distal: beyond.
59   Femoral bifurcation: The dividing point of the main femoral artery into its superficial and deep branches.
60   Femoral crossover bypass: a bypass graft, usually made of prosthetic (artificial) material sewn to both femoral arteries to bring blood from one leg to the other.

wound infection, especially if the examiner has not washed their hands beforehand.

Recognizing that MRSA was also creating havoc for our amputation patients, we introduced the concept of leaving the dressing on for five days, after which the incision could be inspected. By doing so, the amputation wound infection rates fell, although stump revision rates were unchanged, due to patients forgetting they no longer had two legs to stand on and falling, traumatizing the stump.

So, if leaving the dressing on for five days produced better wound results in the most compromised patients on the ward, surely this could be applied to all incisions? Unfortunately, not a chance. It is a time-honoured tradition (I don't know when this started) that surgical residents wake up every patient each morning by ripping off their dressing. Nothing good ever came from that practice but it continues to be done every day and likely in every hospital.

If there is a wound problem, the patient may have a fever, or there could be obvious things about the incision such as profuse drainage, swelling, erythema[61], or pain that would indicate something is happening and the wound should be inspected. On the other hand, if none of those features are present, nothing will be gained by ripping off the dressing. All it does is induce pain for the patient and potentially introduce infection to the incision. Try as I might, I have been completely unsuccessful in teaching residents that "no problem" surgical dressings do not need to be removed daily in order to inspect the underlying incision. Hopefully, one of the readers can continue my effort.

For the patient with proven MRSA, our behaviour (isolation, wearing PPE, plus giving potentially toxic vancomycin) was

---

61   Erythema: redness sometimes signifying inflammation or infection.

necessary for their well-being. Not so, if the patient was a transfer from another hospital or had no wounds. Those patients had swabs taken from their nares[62], axillae[63], and anus. If any one of the swabs came back positive, they were quarantined with all the other MRSA patients and forevermore labelled as *MRSA positive*, even though they might only be a carrier. Some patients with no active clinical problems were thrown into MRSA "dungeons," and developed MRSA wound infections. Whether they were going to develop an MRSA infection or not was unknown. For the ones labelled with the MRSA tag, it could be great if they got a private room; or, it could be horrendous, being confined in a four bed MRSA isolation room. The only way an MRSA carrier could ever be labelled as *clean*, or *no MRSA*, was for them to undergo three consecutive MRSA screening tests and for all of them to come back negative. Not surprisingly, not many patients bothered.

In the end, we adjusted to MRSA by improving our hand hygiene (there are annual awards for the units with the cleanest hands— sadly, the doctors have never won the award), changing our surgical practice (different incisions, use of muscle flaps, antibiotic beads), and changing our admission screening practices. But now we have a host of terrible antibiotic resistant organisms to deal with, such as vancomycin-resistant enterococcus, and toxigenic *Escherichia coli*, to name two. But what we learned, we have applied to these emerging strains of resistant bacteria.

"Our most significant opportunities will be found in times of greatest challenge" (Thomas S. Monson).

62　Nares: nostrils.
63　Axillae: armpits.

11

THE DOWNSIDE TO THE CLOSURE OF
THE VGH NURSING SCHOOL (1998)

"Ginger" (nicknamed for her red hair) was working early Sunday morning at the White Spot Restaurant on West Broadway when I came in with my family for breakfast. Surprised to see her, all I could say was, "What are you doing here?"

"Oh, hi Doc," she said. "Yeah, I've been working here ever since I started on West 8 eighteen months ago. But I'm not alone. All of us full-time grad nurses are working two jobs." When asked why a recent graduate nurse would need to work additional part time elsewhere, she said it was because her full-time nursing salary was inadequate to cover her student loans and living expenses.

Ginger was not a graduate of the VGH School of Nursing. It had closed by 1998, primarily as it was not graduating nurses with a baccalaureate degree—an educational requirement necessary for advancement into nursing administration.

For one hundred years, the VGH nursing school had produced nurses, primarily as low-cost, well-trained labour for the hospital. In return, employment with the hospital served as an early stepping stone for newly graduated nurses. The school recruited students (almost all female) directly from high school and, in exchange for room and board, the student nurses would receive a basic nursing education over three years, and graduate with an RN designation. The instructors were all experienced nurses, most trained in the "VGH way": rounding with the physicians at any time, but not making tea and sandwiches as their colleagues were still doing in other parts of the British Commonwealth.

This VGH way was seen as old-fashioned, or even worse, as if the nurses were the physicians' handmaidens. The new nursing graduates, now armed with their university degrees, were expected to function as independent professionals, to make their own assessments and recommendations. Instead of participating in direct communication with the rounding physicians regarding key patient information, nurses were now frequently unavailable. Instead, all communication was through the patient charts.

This splintering effect of professionals not working closely inevitably leads to poor patient outcomes. This divergent type of health care is seen in every hospital today. On many wards at VGH, there is still the old style of nurses communicating directly with the physicians. But in other hospitals, it is not uncommon for nurses to only communicate with physicians through the patient charts.

A basic goal of hospitals is to treat the sick and discharge them safely, either back home or to a nursing facility. The converse, hospital deaths, can be a measure of how a hospital is performing. The hospital standardized mortality rate (HSMR) is a statistic not widely available to the public but shared amongst hospital administrators across Canada. Collected by the Canadian Institute for Health Information (CIHI), it measures the mortality of hospitalized patients in many hospitals across Canada. It is a comparison of a particular hospital's death rate to the national average. If the hospital's mortality is the same as the national average, then the ratio is 1. If a hospital's death rate is better than the national average, it will be less than 1, and if it is worse, it will be more than 1. The primary reason this data is not widely used as a measurement of hospital performance is it skews the data to make hospitals that have a large hospice function look particularly bad (the HSMR is much greater than 1), as they provide care to the terminally ill.

On the other hand, nobody goes into a hospital for an operation and expects to die from the procedure. So, the HSMR is further divided into the surgical and medical sides of the house. For a national comparison of surgery, one can only measure common operations done in any of the one hundred hospitals CIHI collects data on. These are procedures such as hernia repair, cholecystectomies, hip surgery, etc. Nothing as exotic as vascular or cardiac surgery. In 2007 (the last year that CIHI collected these figures), the HSMR for VGH surgery was 0.66—the best in the country (Canadian Institute for Health Information 2007).

So, what could explain this? It could be the quality of the surgeons and anesthetists, but these are common procedures, and any well-trained physician should have excellent results. I believe it is something about the hospital itself, perhaps being a teaching hospital, but the quality of nursing care cannot be ignored. There may be immeasurable benefits to having nurses regularly round with physicians for improved communication and having designated areas for more intense one-to-one nursing care for extremely ill patients.

In Ginger's case, by the time the VGH School of Nursing was closed, a high school graduate who wanted to pursue a nursing career needed to go to university. There, the student had many choices for a four-year degree program, ranging from the arts to sciences—even engineering. The competition to attract students to the nursing program is fierce. However, room and board are not provided, and many students are forced to take out student loans. The average nurse graduate has $30,000 of student debt the day they qualify, compared with no debt when the nursing school was operating.

Having cost-efficient student nurses also benefited the hospital as there was not the dire continuous nursing shortage we have today. Whichever way we look at it, high quality nursing is vital for patient safety and outcomes. Not all nurses wish to pursue a career in nursing administration, so the insistence of the nursing leaders on requiring all their graduates to have baccalaureate degrees is expensive for the students and for society, because of the nursing shortages created.

As for Ginger, she was recruited by US head-hunters within the year, as were many of her classmates. Canadian universities trained many of the finest nurses, only for them to leave the labour pool. To this day, there have been no further attempts to bring back the nursing schools of bygone years. But, for those who can still remember, there were things that perhaps were done better that have been long discarded.

When children commit errors against others, their parents expect them to apologize and make up. However, when adults commit errors, who asks them to apologize? More importantly, if you have committed a mistake, why can't you admit this and take steps to correct it?

12

THE BARER-STODDART REPORT

It has been said that if you asked any physician who practised in the 1990s why there is a shortage of family physicians, they would say it is was due to the Barer-Stoddart Report. Before discussing the report, one needs to recognize the central role of the federal and provincial governments in the Canadian healthcare system.

The Canadian healthcare system, started in 1964, had the central tenets of being universal, comprehensive, portable, and publicly administered. Although it has served the Canadian public well, issues related to the supply, mix, distribution, regulation, remuneration, and training of physicians had permeated Canadian healthcare policy for at least three decades.

An urgent need for change prompted the cross-Canada Conference of Deputy Ministers of Health (CDMH) in late 1989 to review the potential for regional and national approaches to physician resource policy in Canada. The objective of physician resource policy was to satisfy the physician needs of the population most efficiently, subject to decisions by the population about the resources it was willing to commit to meeting those needs.

To address these issues, the ministers commissioned two health care economists: Morris Barer and Greg Stoddart. Their work was completed the following year and the report released by the CDMH in 1991. Subsequently, this report was published in the Canadian Medical Association Journal in twelve parts from 1992 to 1993 (Barer and Stoddart 1992). Their report stated unequivocally that there was no technically correct or optimum number of physicians (Barer and Stoddart 1992).

The report identified two tiers of problems. The more serious, or first tier, problems included graduates of foreign medical schools, mix and number of residency training positions, role and funding of academic medical centres, poor geographic distribution of physicians, and fee-for-service remuneration. The second tier of problems included undergraduate medical school curricula and postgraduate training exposure, proliferation of subspecialties and residency training programs, licensure, and self-regulation (Barer and Stoddart 1992).

Overall, fifty-three recommendations were made, but the ministers chose to focus on only one of these recommendations, namely the reduction of medical school enrolment to 1600 students for the country. Essentially, this was a 10 percent decrease in enrolment positions at the medical school level as well as a 10 percent reduction of residency training positions. This choice was presumably since the ministers thought it could save money (Evans and McGrail 2008).

This was not the intent of the two authors, who had cautioned against the application of only one or two of these recommendations. They felt that significant change to the supply and mix of Canadian physicians could only occur if all of the guidelines were undertaken in an organized fashion. Nonetheless, this cherry picking led to a lack of physicians five to six years later (Evans and McGrail 2008).

The lack of medical practitioners unleashed a torrent of criticism from those who believed the inability of patients to find a family physician lay at the feet of the Barer-Stoddart report. Critics of the policy used the ratio of the number of physicians to population within Canada over time, and compared it with other countries as indicative of the woefully inadequate number of Canadian physicians, despite Barer-Stoddard's original recommendation against the use of these statistics.

Apart from people's inability to find a family physician (in 2007, 14 percent of Canadians, or five million, were without a family doctor [Esmail 2016]), the other effect of the report was an increased workload for the remaining Canadian physicians, which led to a partial withdrawal of services, especially when it came to being on-call. Previously, it had always been understood that the quid pro quo for admitting privileges to a hospital was taking call pro bono. The only remunerated services were medical services such as consults and procedures while on-call.

However, toward the end of the 1990s, when the full effect of the reduction in medical school enrollments and reductions in residency positions began to be felt throughout the country, the physicians in Prince George, BC were some of the first to reduce services. They refused to work more than a one-in-four on-call schedule. Subsequently, on nights where there was no physician in the community to take call, emergencies would be transferred to the Vancouver hospitals. As a result, this led to the larger Vancouver teaching hospitals being inundated with transfer patients. Things got so bad, there was public discussion about whether patients would need to be transferred out of province (to Alberta) or out of country (to Seattle) to receive care.

The government's response was to pay the Prince George physicians to be on-call. However, once an on-call stipend was satisfactorily negotiated, each surrounding medical community, not surprisingly, also demanded to be paid to be on-call. Being at the end of the supply and demand chain, the government continued to pay on-call stipends. The requirement to now be paid to be on-call spread like wildfire throughout the province. From there, it extended to several other provinces. Once physicians were accustomed to being paid to be on-call, there was no going back; since then all physicians are paid to be on-call. The only difference is the payment amount—physicians whose call may be very intensive (Tier 1 or Call Group A) are paid at a higher rate than those physicians whose call is less intensive.

After five years of contraction, medical schools throughout Canada have been ramping up. Currently, approximately 2,500 students graduate from Canadian medical schools annually (in 1990, at the beginning of the Barer-Stoddart report, there were approximately 1,800 annual graduates). Despite the rapid increase in medical graduates (which outpaces population growth), the issue of inadequate family physicians has not been addressed. Pundits may blame this on the Barer-Stoddart report, but it could well be for other reasons such as the dissolution of the rotating internship program (see "Who Killed Rotating Internship?"), or an overall reduction in (family practice) medical services. Part of this may be related to subspecialization, and part of it may be related to the feminization of medicine (approximately 70 percent of medical school graduates are now female). On average, women put in less time than men over a career (Evans and McGrail 2008). Another possibility is that current young physicians have different career expectations than their predecessors. The current medical student selection process tries to choose candidates with life experience in addition to high grades. Although these candidates may become excellent physicians, whether their work ethic will match their predecessors appears to be unlikely (Evans and McGrail 2008).

If physicians do not provide adequate medical services, it allows for the intrusion of non-physician groups to do so. Already, nurse practitioners have been assuming this role in physician-starved areas, although whether they are as effective as physicians is uncertain (Patrick 2000).

The issue of both Canadian and non-Canadian foreign medical graduates has also never been adequately addressed. Many are currently unemployed as physicians, while waiting for a residency position. This uncoordinated policy wastes the benefits of overseas training facilities and the distribution of physicians in underserved communities (Barer and Stoddart 1992). Recently, due to the introduction of competency-based education, resident physician shortages amongst the teaching hospitals has led to discussions allowing foreign medical graduates clinical associate positions in hospitals funded by the health regions.

The unresolved issues of physician availability, maldistribution, and remuneration will remain contentious (Stoddart and Barer 1999). By failing to respond to the Barer-Stoddart report in an organized and comprehensive way, an over-abundance of physicians in already heavily serviced areas, providing more medical services despite a continual lack of available family physicians in both the rural and urban areas, will undoubtedly lead to future discrepancies between physician payments and service received. In short, the

Canadian federal and provincial governments and Canadian public will likely end up paying more while receiving less.

> *"The easiest thing in the world is to do nothing. I hope you do not do what is easy..." (Barak Obama)*

13

Vascular Surgery 2001

As a result of the Barer-Stoddart report, a strategic planning committee of the UBC Division of Vascular Surgery was formed in 1992, chaired by Henry Litherland, to determine vascular surgeon levels required to maintain academic standards in the UBC teaching hospitals while accommodating BC's requirement for vascular surgery services.

In the early 1990s, planning was being conducted by everybody from the Divisions, Departments, and even the University. The latter had created a university-wide planning committee, the Council of University Teaching Hospitals (COUTH), to develop or improve programs. In order to achieve this, COUTH was struck to consider movement of different disciplines to leverage the talents of individuals throughout the city as well as the strengths of the institutions. After much consideration, for Surgery, COUTH recommended the transfer of St. Paul's neurosurgery to VGH in return for transferring part of the cardiac surgery program at VGH to St. Paul's as the latter was to be designated the Cardiac Centre. Although the move was welcomed by (VGH) neurosurgery, the loss of neurosurgery from SPH led to its downgrade as a major trauma hospital. Vascular surgery was also considered for amalgamation completely at the VGH site, but this was quickly shot down.

The chief goal for the strategic planning committee was to address recommendation #27 of the Barer-Stoddart report that "the academic medicine establishment should show more leadership in several important areas, including: adapting the training of physicians to changing social needs, monitoring the supply and mix of physicians and the appropriateness of the services they provide, maintaining a balance among different types of research, and contributing to more effective continuing education and competency assurance programmes" (Barer and Stoddart 1991).

The UBC Division of Vascular Surgery committee, consisting of members from academia and the community, was tasked with reviewing the definition of a vascular surgeon, the services provided by a vascular surgeon (including academic services), the current population and volume of clinical services, the current resources to provide surgical services, the current resources available for surgeon services, and the projections for future resource utilization, volume of services, and resources for vascular surgery services.

The second purpose of the committee was to respond to the 1991 report by the Royal Commission on Health Care and Costs entitled, "Closer to Home." British Columbia, like much of Canada, is a vast under-populated province. Residents who develop major illnesses require the services of highly trained specialists and need to travel long distances for their care. Siding with the cries of patients and their families from the smaller communities rather than the physicians, the Commission recommended that wherever possible, health care should be available in the smaller communities.

The committee defined a vascular surgeon as a surgeon who had completed their fellowship requirements in general and vascular surgery and provided vascular surgical services full time. Based on an assumption that the volume of clinical services would be proportional to the population, they used an estimate of 1 full-time surgeon for 55,000 persons aged 44 or older. Using these criteria, there were 10 vascular surgeons in the COUTH hospitals and 32 (13 fulltime and 19 part time) surgeons who provided vascular surgery services in the community hospitals. The 32 included general, as well as cardiothoracic, surgeons.

In order to satisfy the Royal Commission's "Closer to Home" document, the human resource projection recommended that by 2001 there should be 8 vascular surgeons in the COUTH hospitals—a reduction of 2 surgeons, since fewer patients will need to be transferred to the teaching hospitals, and there should be 38 full and part-time vascular surgeons for the community hospitals. Other considerations, such as support staff, radiology suites, and diagnostic vascular labs were also projected to increase, although no figures were given for those.

Not surprisingly, none of the recommendations were taken. What has happened since is summarized in the following table:

Year	BC Population > 44 years	# vasc surgeons		Population served/ surgeon	
		UBC	non-COUTH		
1992	1,066,364	10	32	25,389	
2001	1,131,259	8	38	24,592	(projected)
2016	1,738,157	9	21	57,938	(actual)

Table 1. Comparison of BC population and vascular surgeons over time.

In 1992, there were 42 vascular surgeons practising in BC, of which 23 were full time. Ten of the full-time surgeons worked in the teaching or COUTH hospitals and 32 worked in the community or non-COUTH hospitals. Each surgeon served a population of around 25,000 (based on need for major arterial surgery).

In order to keep patients closer to home without eroding academic output, Litherland's recommendation was for 8 COUTH surgeons (2 less than in 1992) and 38 (6 more than in 1992) non-COUTH surgeons by 2001.

In reality, by 2016, the BC population greater than 44 years (the group most likely to need vascular surgery services), had increased 63 percent, from 1,066,364 to 1,738,157. By that time, there were no more surgeons doing part time vascular surgery. However, the total number of vascular surgeons throughout BC was fewer than in 1992. By 2016, there were 9 in the COUTH hospitals and 21 in the community, or non-COUTH hospitals. Each surgeon was responsible for 57,938 patients. The reasons for this reduction are complex, owing to factors of available hospital resources and overall health care funding. With more patients to look after with the same or dwindling resources, waiting lists could only go up.

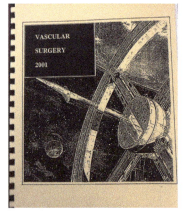

Dr. Litherland's conclusions were presented in a document titled "Vascular Surgery 2001." It was one of the first times a comprehensive examination of manpower needs in Canada was conducted. Although the recommendations were ignored, the process of collecting and analyzing the information is the legacy that Dr. Litherland has left for us (Litherland 1993).

14

Hickman Lines -
The Second Skirmish with Radiology

Of all things to disagree about, why would you pick a fight over the least glamorous of procedures? Turf wars are common in medicine, as elsewhere in society. Amongst surgical specialties, the general surgeons compete with the ENT (Ear, Nose, and Throat) surgeons over head and neck tumours, the plastic surgeons compete with the ENT surgeons over faces and noses, and the cardiac and vascular surgeons disagree on who should look after thoracic aortic cases. One thing these turf wars have in common is that the disease they are competing for is "sexy," or a large problem.

At other times, it appears the reason for the intense competition is because a procedure is highly lucrative. A glaring example of this is the treatment of varicose veins. In the unregulated US, lack of a specific fellowship does not mean you cannot work in that area. Practitioners who treat venous disorders are numerous, ranging from family doctors, phlebologists[64], dermatologists, vascular sur-

---

64   Phlebologists: physicians who specialise in vein treatments.

geons, and even interested gynecologists, and the list goes on and on. Where there is (big) money to be made, it attracts a pack.

But, Hickman lines? Why would anybody want to scrap over that? A Hickman line is a tunnelled central venous catheter, adapted by Dr. R. Hickman (Hickman et al. 1979), a nephrologist in Seattle, from the original central venous catheter developed by Dr. J. Broviac (Broviac, Cole, Scribner 1973). Having one, two, or three lumens[65], they were designed for long-term chemotherapy but could also be used for long term infusion for parenteral nutrition[66] or antimicrobials. Tunnelled central venous catheters have also been modified for dialysis (Permcath) and may be a completely closed port with one or two lumens (portocath).

As the vascular fellow, I never did any of these procedures, feeling that they were "beneath me." At the time, all Hickman lines were done by Dr. Tony Salvian and a general surgeon, Dr. Greg McGregor. They seemed tedious enough. All procedures were done in the operating room, usually at the end of a slate or as an emergency. Patients were sedated, and using local anesthetic, two incisions were made: one, either in the neck over the external jugular vein, or in the deltopectoral groove[67] for the cephalic vein; the catheter would exit through a second incision in the anterior chest, inferior to the first incision. These cases typically took between thirty to forty-five minutes to complete. Through technical improvements with ultrasound-guided punctures of the internal jugular or subclavian veins and specially designed kits containing the tunnelling devices, these procedures now usually take no more than fifteen minutes.

---

65 Lumens: openings.
66 Parenteral nutrition: intravenous nutrition.
67 Deltopectoral groove: soft tissue space below the collar bone and medial to the shoulder.

In my first year of practice, I realized I should have paid more attention to these simplest of procedures. Although by then, I had done lots of pacemakers by cutting down on the cephalic vein in the deltopectoral groove, I encountered a particularly challenging case. The patient had acute leukemia and needed a Hickman line for chemotherapy. However, her platelet count was only 12 x 10^9/L (normal is 150–400 x 10^9/L). Even though she received platelet transfusions pre-procedure, the continuous oozing made exposure very tedious. After flailing for two hours the case was finally finished. For my effort, I was paid around $300. That day I learned that there were "...Hickman line patients and then there were other Hickman line patients..."

With the boom in bone marrow transplantation and long-term chemotherapy for many different tumours, the need for central venous access continued to grow. The VGH vascular surgery service performed around 600 Hickman line cases of various types annually. But these cases were done at inopportune times, frequently at night and on weekends, since there was no dedicated time in the operating room. Nonetheless, with these large annual volumes, even though the cases paid very little, jokes were made about "the house built from Hickman lines."

Those "good" times were about to end when, in the 1990s, the radiologists wanted a piece of the action. On his return to Vancouver, an interventional radiologist[68] who had practised in Ontario where the interventional radiology service received direct referrals from all physicians, rather than just vascular surgeons, felt that radiology should increase their volumes by doing venous access procedures.

68   Interventional radiologist: Radiologists diagnose disease based on imaging (X-ray, CT, MRI). Interventional radiologists are those radiologists who also do procedures using imaging techniques.

When this became apparent, our response was to outcompete the radiologists.

As a result, we spent the next few years dragging our weary bodies in the middle of the night to do these cases. This drove the operating room crazy. They could not understand why we would use such valuable resources to perform these minor procedures in the middle of the night. In response, they created a large closet-sized room on the outskirts of the main operating rooms for these procedures. We struggled in this fashion for a few more years before we were thrown a life preserver. The interventional cardiologists had a brand new cath lab[69] they could not fill with sufficient cases to keep their staff numbers up. Besides, the OR at this point was disgusted that we continued to do these minor procedures in the main operating room. So out we went.

Time in the cath lab was paradise. Here we were surrounded by like-minded health care professionals who were equally motivated to do procedures efficiently. The only problem was their procedure table, which could not tilt to place patients in a reverse Trendelenburg position. Not surprisingly, our pneumothorax[70] rate was as high as 10 percent if we had to blindly puncture the subclavian or internal jugular veins based on surface landmarks. This significant patient morbidity lead to a change in practice. We adapted and learned how to use intraoperative ultrasound and perform ultrasound-guided percutaneous procedures. Around the same time, the introduction of specific device kits simplified the procedure even further; we could safely and efficiently complete a procedure within fifteen to twenty minutes.

---

69   Cath lab: abbreviated from *catheter laboratory*. This is the area where interventional cardiologists do procedures such as coronary stents.
70   Pneumothorax: lung collapse.

After several more years of working in the cath lab, a truce was negotiated with the radiologists such that we would jointly do Hickman lines and other venous access procedures in the radiology suite. The interventional cardiologists at this point were also highly motivated to see us depart, as the rush of new interventional cardiology procedures was starting to boom.

Currently, central venous access procedures are performed by both radiologists and vascular surgeons on a daily basis in the radiology suite. These procedures have been dramatically simplified with the addition of ultrasound and specific device kits. As we have mastered this now even simpler technique, we primarily use these as teaching sessions for the junior residents and medical students.

What initially was an attempt to prevent a hostile takeover turned out to be an excellent example of what can be accomplished with compromise and diplomacy.

15

—

THE HONG KONG CONNECTION

In 1998, I was recommended by my department head, Dr. Richard Finley, to be a visiting speaker at the annual Hong Kong Surgical Forum. The latter was the brainchild of Professors John Wong and G. B. Ong. Each year, the University of Hong Kong invites three or four visiting speakers. I had the good fortune of talking about vascular surgery and my primary research interest at that time, photo-dynamic therapy for vascular diseases. The forum lasted three days, after which we were flown to Shanghai, China, to give the same talks to Mainland Chinese surgeons.

Being in Hong Kong, presenting at the forum, and meeting all the staff at Hong Kong University (HKU) opened my eyes to how great collaboration could still happen with only a small investment. At the time, the Vascular Surgery Division at HKU was very small and essentially run by Dr. Stephen Cheng. But the setup, with their vascular lab being adjacent to the ward, and Stephen's dedication to creating a comprehensive database from the very first patient, was truly impressive. The database contained demographics, hematology and biochemistry results, indications for surgery, procedures performed, outcomes, plus imaging results for every patient operated on. When patients came back to the clinic, long term follow-up data would be added. That commitment to create and maintain a comprehensive database has been the basis of multiple publications that have come from their division. It was an impressive demonstration that you do not need to be from a large institution with lots of patients in order to publish interesting results. Being from a smaller institution but meticulously documenting the results with excellent follow-up could also generate many high-quality publications.

Stephen and I became fast friends and to cement the relationship between UBC and HKU, we cross-trained a number of trainees. Jerry Chen, having recently completed his vascular fellowship, was sent to Harbor-UCLA and then to the HKU for additional training in 1998.

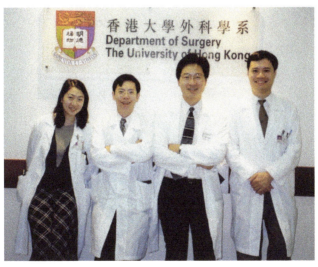

Starting something great.
Left to right: Jennifer Sihoe, Albert Ting, Jerry Chen, Stephen Cheng. c. 1998.

In return, HKU sent four fellows to train at UBC: Albert Ting, Arthur Chan, Edward Hui, and Rennie Yien. Each of them was unique. They were serious but could be outrageously funny when the situation-called for it. The education, however, was not one-sided. They taught us a number of things, such as managing MRSA patients (see "When MRSA Came to Town") and, thanks to watching Rennie Yien, how to expertly use a nerve hook to tighten sutures.

This relationship with HKU was strengthened when we invited Stephen Cheng to be a visiting professor the same year. Since then, I have been back to Hong Kong as visiting professor six times, at the invitation of HKU or the Chinese University of Hong Kong, together with the Hong Kong Hospital Authority, to teach Evidence-Based Surgery. It was during these professorships that I learned some cultural nuances. In North America, open discussion between student and teacher, as well as the entire class, is encouraged. This helps clear up misconceptions and keeps students on their toes. In Hong Kong, however, although we were told the students were very smart, you wouldn't know since none of them asked questions. This is a cultural difference, and reflects how the students show respect for the teacher. However, I got around this issue with food by insisting on having lunch with the students. After lunch, the students were fully engaged with lots of questions, and, yes, they were very smart.

Surgeons and institutions need cross fertilization. We should actively encourage exchanges to gain an understanding of how surgeons work and think in different parts of the world. The creation of the Hong Kong Surgical Forum, with generous sponsorship, was pure genius. Given a limited or even non-existent budget (except for sponsorship), experts can be invited, friendships established, and reciprocities extended to enhance understanding. No matter where we are, the same issues always come up. I have seen the same type of genius thinking behind another vascular surgery meeting, the Vascular International Padova, established by Professor Franco Grego at the University of Padova. Calling it *a meeting of friends*, the biannual meeting is a must for me to see friends from all over the world. At UBC, we have invited a number of key vascular surgeons to be visiting professors or reviewers, from Drs. Jimmy Yao, Eugene Strandness, Rodney White, Joe Mills, Jeff Ballard, Peter Schneider, Michel Makaroun, Wayne Johnston, Tom Lindsay, Tom Forbes, Randy Guzman, Kaj Johansen, Ben Starnes, Omid Jazaeri, and Sherene Shahlub. With each invitee, new ideas are discussed, future collaborations are proposed, and greater understanding is achieved. This needs to continue. If residents are the lifeline for the program, then visiting professors are the lighthouses.

No money! That's not a problem. But no ideas? Now that's a problem.

PART FOUR

THE JIM PATTISON TOWER YEARS

(2003–PRESENT)

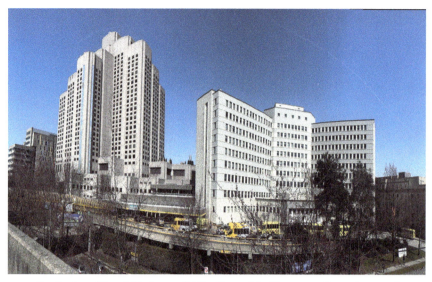

Jim Pattison (L) and Blackmore (R) Pavilions of the Vancouver General Hospital

In the late 1980s, a third tower—the Laurel Pavilion—was planned at VGH. By 1996, the first three floors were open but none of these floors contained patient wards. After sitting empty for many years, a generous donor who had been a patient at VGH, billionaire Jim Pattison, pledged to fund the completion of the Laurel Pavilion provided the provincial government would match his donation. With the increased funds, the new pavilion was opened in 2003 and named after its largest donor.

There was a consequence to this, however. Prior to the completion of the tower, VGH had long been unofficially recognized as the dominant hospital for the province by physicians and the populace. As it also had the largest budget for all BC hospitals, its CEO, the outstanding Murray Martin, was frequently in the news regarding health care issues. A requirement for provincial funding to complete the pavilion was the sacking of the VGH CEO. Soon after, not only was a new CEO chosen, but the concept of regionalization was introduced.

VGH became part of Vancouver Coastal Health, a massive region representing not just Vancouver, but also Richmond, and communities up the Sunshine Coast. The VGH CEO was now the leader of the new region, and with stakeholders from all of the communities represented, the "power" of VGH was diluted as the interests of the smaller communities were also considered. The "Big House" was no longer (Marty McLoughlin, personal communication).

For vascular surgery, the UBCH surgeons were merged with the VGH surgeons to make one large group. The enlarged group moved from the Centennial Pavilion into the Jim Pattison Pavilion (Tower 8) in 2003. However, the resources, including beds and OR time, were not fully transferred to VGH—a victim of the merger to make UBCH a dedicated outpatient surgery and medical clinics facility.

16

Bringing Endovascular to VGH

Although use of balloon angioplasty and stents to treat vascular disease had been described in the 1960s and 1980s, respectively, these outpatient-based endovascular procedures were relegated to the interventional radiologists for the treatment of short lesions[71], primarily in the iliac arteries. Vascular surgeons were generally not interested in these less invasive procedures.

In 1991, however, the most disruptive technology to impact the future of vascular surgery was described by Dr. Juan Parodi, an Argentinian (Parodi, Palmaz, Barone 1991). Parodi showed that aortic aneurysms could be treated by re-lining the interior of the aneurysms using covered stents, thereby excluding the aneurysms from the luminal blood. Parodi had conceptualized his idea while observing the physiologic insult of open aortic surgery as a surgical trainee at the Cleveland Clinic.

His paper describing this technique was met with extreme skepticism. The premier vascular surgery journal, the *Journal of Vascular Surgery,* refused to publish his findings. Consequently, Parodi could only publish it in a less impactful journal, the *Annals of Vascular*

---

71 Short lesions: atherosclerotic plaques usually less than 2 cm in length.

Surgery. This seminal piece of work, though, is now the most highly cited reference in our specialty (ibid.).

The importance of this paper was not lost on the editor, the late Dr. John Bergan, who wrote in his editorial commentary, ". . .opposition to the procedure will be mounted. In Vascular Surgery no change for the better has occurred that wise and good men have not opposed . . . "

Bergan's prediction of opposition was prescient. This new technology seemed to have limited scope to treat the variety of different anatomic variants. Nonetheless, many centres started to adopt this new technology, including UBCH. In 1997, Peter Fry and Lindsay Machan performed the first endovascular aneurysm repair (EVAR) in Canada.

Despite the initial adoption of EVAR to treat AAAs, the teaching of this technique to faculty and new trainees was not organized. Initially, there were no training courses available. Surgical trainees were there to provide initial groin cutdown and femoral artery exposure, and subsequent groin closure at the end of the case. There were no opportunities to learn wire skills or graft deployment. Those filling this type of limited role would later be sarcastically described as "can openers."

When it became obvious that this may be the future for vascular surgery, I decided to take a sabbatical and educate myself in endovascular surgery. From our experience with transplantation, doing nothing would mean being pushed aside and letting others do the work we had previously done for years. However, there were huge obstacles. First, nobody from our group had ever gone on sabbatical. To go on one would be a major expense in terms of lost income and on-going expenses. Second, where would one go? There was no training centre in Canada. There were only rumours of training sites throughout the world. I approached Interventional Radiology (IR) wishing to be trained in endovascular but received a chilly reception. Prior to this, we had been collegial in sending angioplasty cases to IR when we thought they could be done without open surgery, with the understanding that surgical backup was available should the case need immediate surgical correction. The consistent message I received was that, as surgeons, we had nothing to offer the radiologists, and our skill set could never match theirs.

Undaunted, I visited a number of locations, including Toronto, Calgary, Honolulu, and Milan, but it was only after visiting Dr. Ron Dalman at Stanford in 2003 did a path appear. Ron told me of an opportunity in Lubbock, Texas for vascular surgeons to train with Dr. Michael Silva, one of the few willing to train vascular surgeons in a three-month endovascular fellowship position. In fact, Ron had already signed up and was leaving to train under Mike.

After contacting Mike Silva, and making preparatory arrangements to go to Lubbock, Mike took up a new position as chief of Vascular Surgery at the Cleveland Clinic. So, my plans again changed, and I started to complete new paperwork to spend my fellowship at the Cleveland Clinic.

Jerry Chen, then our youngest member of staff, had the same realization that endovascular was the future of our specialty. He sought an endovascular fellowship in Pittsburgh under Dr. Michel Makaroun, also in the same year, 2006. Our plan was for two of the four surgeons at VGH to be formally trained in endovascular and that the others, David Taylor and Tony Salvian, would learn the art through osmosis when we returned. Afterwards, any new appointee taken on at VGH would require additional training in endovascular.

Financially, both of us took it on the chin. After we returned, we approached IR about a shared workload and teaching responsibilities. Again, they were not interested and thus, Jerry and I did all of our endovascular procedures together in the operating room. In order to gain experience quickly, we "double scrubbed" on every case, realizing that financially, this was another loss leader. The radiologists criticized our technique and introduced the documentation of how much fluoroscopy[72] time we used on each procedure in their reports, although previously, for their procedures, there was no mention of fluoroscopy time.

Fortunately, we had no major complications, our procedures became more efficient, and we started to train our trainees. Patients also benefited, as any complication that arose during the procedure would be corrected either by endovascular or open surgical means. With more experience from complicated cases, the addition of Drs. Joel Gagnon and Keith Baxter, and independence from the interventional radiologists, the vascular surgeons became the recognized endovascular experts.

Two other requirements for endovascular management deserve special mention. These are the devices required and the OR nursing staff.

Prior to endovascular procedures, our prosthetic budget was minuscule. The most expensive device we used was a PTFE graft, costing around $2000 per graft, but at that time, we were allowed to re-sterilize whatever uncontaminated piece was not used. Endovascular is very expensive with its array of disposables: wires, catheters, stents, and grafts. Acquiring these devices required convincing the hospital that, in the future, ruptured AAAs would

72   Fluoroscopy: X-ray imaging.

be done endovascularly in the OR, as there were a number of preliminary reports showing improved patient survival compared with open surgery. Thus, readily available supplies to handle these cases were needed, which would require expanding the budget from several thousand to over a million dollars annually. We (along with Anesthesia and IR) successfully convinced the hospital. For their collaborative role in this joint program, our division is indebted to two individuals, Dr. Mike Martin from Radiology and Dr. Andrew Sawka from Anesthesia.

Since Radiology was not interested in sharing expertise, this also meant they were against the idea of sharing staff. The training of OR nurses who would be competent in this new paradigm would again fall to the surgeons. Dedicated training sessions were established and to this day, every few months, a new group of OR nurses rotate through vascular surgery, learning these new techniques. It is not ideal, but it has worked for us.

We finally learned from our inaction regarding our role in transplantation that if you really want something, you have to go out and get it. It will be hard, and you will struggle. Nobody is going to gift-wrap and hand it to you. The alternative is to do nothing, but that only breeds mediocrity.

17

CHAOULLI VERSUS QUEBEC

Being on the west coast of Canada, we were stunned by the results of the Chaoulli case in 2005. This was a landmark case that tested one of the key pillars of the Canadian Health Care system and threatened to tear apart the publicly funded system.

The Chaoulli case was based on a seventy-three-year-old Quebecer, George Zeliotis, who suffered from a number of health ailments, including hip problems. He was scheduled for hip replacement surgery, but when the wait time for his procedure became excessive, he became an advocate for reducing wait times in Quebec. In particular, Zeliotis argued that if the public health care system could not provide care in a timely way, then citizens of Quebec should have the option of paying to have their care expedited. Dr. Jacques Chaoulli was a physician who provided home appointments. After being denied a licence to open an independent private hospital, he joined Zeliotis to contest the prohibition of private medical insurance in the province of Quebec.

The case made its way to the Supreme Court of Canada and in a narrow 4-3 decision the Court found that the Quebec Health Insurance Act and Hospital Insurance Act, that prohibited private medical insurance despite long waiting lists, violated Quebecers' right to life and security. However, on the ruling whether there was also violation of the Canadian Charter of Rights and Freedoms, the decision was 3-3, so the Chaoulli decision only applied to Quebec (Flood and Sullivan 2005).

As the landmark ruling potentially threatened the Canadian health system, the Attorney General of Quebec asked the Court to suspend its judgment for eighteen months. The court instead granted only a twelve-month suspension, to expire in June 2006.

The response in BC was swift. That the Chaoulli case applied only in Quebec and the court's action was suspended for twelve months meant that all of the other Canadian provinces had twelve months to clean up their waiting list; otherwise, there would be a number of similar challenges throughout the rest of Canada. Since the original plaintiff, Zeliotis, suffered from an orthopedic ailment, the province decided to address the orthopedic waiting list problem first. UBCH, now that vascular surgery had left in 2003 along with other services, had been converted to a smaller hospital with primarily medical clinics, a small emergency room, and expanded day surgery. To address the long orthopedic waiting lists, the operating rooms of UBCH increased the orthopedic OR time (at the expense of other services) and developed more efficient ways of managing OR resources, such as use of swing (staggered) rooms to have greater throughput. And to shorten the waiting lists of all orthopedic surgeons throughout the province, any orthopedic surgeon could refer their cases to the Vancouver group or could travel to Vancouver and operate on their patients at UBCH.

This action, not surprisingly, impacted all other services. For vascular surgery, our day surgery OR time became less and less, to the point that my patients' wait time to have minor varicose vein surgery was three years! After the ramp up for orthopedic surgery, other services, from ophthalmology to cardiac surgery, also had increases in their OR resources. Years later, only when a provincial election in the same year was imminent, was there an aggressive attempt to clean up the varicose vein waiting list. For a brief moment in 2014, we had the luxury of seemingly unlimited OR resources to deal with our chronic waiting list problem. But by then waiting lists in Canada were well-politicized.

The Canada Health Act (1984) established a list of conditions (or pillars) for provinces to provide in order to receive their share of federal transfer payments. Provincial health care plans needed to be comprehensive, universal, portable, accessible, and publicly administered. The intent of this act was to provide equal and reasonable health care to all Canadians, including those who had no ability to pay (CMAJ 2005). However, there were criticisms of the act in that it was not comprehensive by not covering abortion, dental, or podiatric care. And it produced waiting lists.

It was the accessible pillar that was contested in the Chaoulli case. Just prior to the Chaoulli verdict, a national strategy, the 2004 Health Accord, was created to address public concerns about the Canadian health system, especially wait times: waiting to see a family physician, waiting for surgery, and waiting in emergency rooms. This was a ten-year federal investment; the total amount was $41 billion. An institution, the Health Council of Canada, was created to monitor it. But in the eighth and final bulletin of the Council, it stated that the improvement "has been modest and Canada's overall performance is lagging behind that of many other high-income countries" (Simpson 2014).

The Health Accord also spawned the Wait Time Alliance, which reported on Canada's wait time progress. It used mathematical and statistical approaches and adopted process improvement methods to reduce wait times (Wait Time Alliance Report Card 2015). But how did it get the original data as to how long is too long to wait?

In vascular surgery, we are fortunate in that many of the diseases we treat, and our procedures, have "hard end points," thus making it easier to measure and compare results. For example, based on the NASCET[73] results, the risk of stroke after a TIA or minor stroke was about 1% per week for 4 weeks. Comparatively, the perioperative stroke or death risk in patients undergoing carotid endarterectomy in the NASCET study was 2% (NASCET 1991). These results were also confirmed in the European carotid study trial (ECST 1991).

Based on this data, patients waiting for more than two weeks to have carotid surgery following a TIA or minor stroke had a higher stroke risk than having surgery during the same time. Thus, the wait time for surgery for a symptomatic carotid stenosis should be no more than two weeks. Using the available literature on the natural history of disease and our surgical results, appropriate wait times could also be constructed for patients with AAA, asymptomatic carotid disease, and critical limb ischemia. On the other hand, the data was less robust for conditions such as failing bypass grafts, dialysis access, and procedures for lifestyle disability. Our group reported the wait times for various procedures, and the percentage of time we were within the waiting period, five years before the Wait Time Alliance was established (Turnbull et al. 2000).

---

73   NASCET: North American Symptomatic Carotid Endarterectomy Trial. A landmark study comparing carotid endarterectomy with medical treatment in patients with transient ischemic attacks (TIA) and carotid artery narrowing.

Although we may have robust data, how do other groups, where the end points are not "hard," but "soft" (such as decreased pain, greater mobility, etc.), determine wait times for their procedures? Where there is no reliable data available (and this may be the case for many specialties), there could be a number of different methods to determine wait times, from patient-focused groups, to simply measuring the current wait times and deeming a percentage, say, 70 percent, to be the "benchmark" wait time. In short, these are all estimates. Based on these estimates, the Wait Time Alliance published their benchmarks for treatment in five categories: cardiac procedures, cancer treatment, diagnostic imaging, joint replacement, and sight restoration in 2005 (Eggerton 2005). By 2015, there were measurements of wait times in sixteen categories, although the measured benefits were still typically modest.

If anything, the data on wait times for surgery may be more optimistic than at first glance. In practice, the clock measuring the wait time for surgery starts once the surgical booking slip is submitted (in paper or electronic form) to the OR booking clerk. Each booking needs to have the procedure code, consent, consult, ECG, imaging, and bloodwork results. For procedures where the wait times are already long, the standard practice at VGH is that the bookings will be returned and asked to be refreshed if the patient has been on the waiting list for more than six months. This work then falls on the surgical secretaries. In order to not have to bring the patient back for a new consult, a new ECG, and new bloodwork, secretaries may simply hang on to the surgical bookings until the patient's name is at the top of the list (Roz Chung, personal communication). Despite verbal admonitions to not do this in order to have accurate data, many secretaries choose to submit their OR booking package much closer to the anticipated date of surgery. Knowing this, of the $41 billion spent on the Health Accord, perhaps some consideration for a "finder's fee" should have been given to the secretaries to get their buy-in?

Today, long waiting lists for patients to see family physicians, see specialists, have diagnostic imaging, and undergo procedures continues. Having an aging population and limited health care resources only worsens the wait time situation. There is still no private health insurance outside of Quebec, although the potential for this may change with future court challenges.

18

Time Out

One of the hardest things to change is physician behaviour. Even when presented with evidence based on published randomized clinical trials, physician behaviour remains difficult to change. The usual thinking is: if one is getting satisfactory results with tried and true methods, then why change? Most physicians only change behaviour based on an N of 1[74]. Every one of us can probably recall the moment we decided to change.

Physician behaviour can also change, not necessarily because of high quality evidence but most certainly due to administrative pressures. Some administrative pressures, such as the need to change into dedicated OR shoes when working in the operating room, were constantly requested of us, but not always adhered to.

The most dramatic change in operating room behaviour occurred in 2010, based on a paper published in the *New England Journal of Medicine* in the preceding year. The lead author, Atul Gawande, a general surgeon from the Brigham Hospital at Harvard had previously written about the risks of surgery. Using a 19-item surgical safety checklist recommended by the World Health Organization,

---

74   N of 1: A clinical trial involving only one patient.

they showed in a non-randomized cohort study from eight hospitals throughout the world (four from industrialized countries and four from developing countries) that, overall, mortality was reduced from 1.5 to 0.8% (p=0.003), and major complications reduced from 11.0 to 7.0% (p<0.001) after introduction of the checklist (Haynes et al. 2009).

Because of the significant benefits demonstrated and the simplicity of the checklist, it was rapidly adopted. Where there was dissension, it was rapidly suppressed with comments such as: "Everybody needs to get behind this; patients are dying," or "This is what the WHO recommends." Almost overnight, checklists were brought in, based on the original 19-item list. Nurses were primarily charged with administering the checklists. Each time a checklist was to be performed, a "time out" was called. These were found to be so simple and so powerful that the original single pre-op checklist was expanded to four checkpoints: there was a pre-surgical huddle at least thirty minutes before each case, a time out as soon as the patient entered the OR, another time out just prior to the procedure starting, and a post-procedure review to see if there was any deviation. Protocols were drawn and attached to each OR, forms were printed in order to check off the boxes, and data was entered: who recorded the data, when it was recorded, and the details.

What was not reviewed was the actual data from the original study. Amongst the four hospitals from industrialized countries, one was from Canada, namely the Toronto General Hospital. Each hospital was expected to recruit five hundred patients over a three-month period. From the results, significant improvements in mortality occurred in only two of the eight hospitals and complications were significantly less in only three of the eight hospitals. The authors, however, did not unblind the specific hospitals nor make reference to which hospitals the safety checklist made no difference. Only by combining the overwhelmingly improved results with the non-significant results was there a measurable significant improvement.

I thought the administrators were zealots blinded by a publication in the *New England Journal of Medicine*. You were either on board with the groupthink or an obstacle in the path of progress. During all my years, I have only encountered one patient who ever made me consider which side we were operating on. It was a carotid patient who was anesthetized before I saw him immediately pre-op. Fortunately my notes and imaging studies confirmed the same side. After that, I made it a point of seeing every patient before they were anesthetized and asking one of the most important questions: Which side are we doing? Like many other surgeons, I made it a point, long before time outs were introduced, to personally review every patient's medication and allergy history, as well as pre-operative antibiotics. Apart from that one episode, the only benefit I have found with time outs is that I got to learn the names of a lot of nurses and anesthetists, as it is a requirement to introduce everybody during the time out.

Once the wheels were set in motion, however, nothing was going to slow down time outs, let alone make them stop. Like many things that become ingrained after three months, this then became behaviour, regardless of whether it makes a difference. In particular, there was never an evaluation plan to see if this time-requiring effort made any difference.

Four years later, a report from Ontario addressing exactly this issue was published. Unlike the previous study, which required approximately five hundred cases from each of the eight hospitals, this was a three-month study examining the outcomes of death and major complications from Ontario hospitals that had a surgical safety checklist program. A total of 101 hospitals participated and contributed 109,341 and 106,370 procedures, respectively, for the three months prior to and three months following the introduction of a surgical safety checklist. The adjusted risk of death at 30 days was 0.71% prior to and 0.65% following the introduction of the surgical safety checklist (p=0.13). Similarly, the risk of surgical complications was 3.86% prior to and 3.82% following implementation of the surgical checklist (p=0.29) (Urbach et al. 2014).

Despite publishing in the *New England Journal of Medicine*, and carefully analyzing the results of more than 100,000 patients (compared with less than 4000 patients from the original study), and most importantly, being a Canadian study, the Urbach study showed that in the province of Ontario, the introduction of time outs made no difference to perioperative death and major complications. So, did it change the behaviour in our hospital? Absolutely not. By now, with a heavy administrative presence bearing down on the surgeons to turn up for the pre-op huddle and come immediately to the OR for the time out, nothing was going to change this new behaviour. The closest we got to discussing it was at a journal club, where one of the surgeons vehemently condemned the Ontario study as being anti-everything. Even the authors of the Ontario study suggested that this should be resolved with a randomized controlled study. So, is there a chance this will happen? Sadly, I suspect not. We will continue this and other types of behaviours despite (or in spite of) the (lack of) evidence.

19

ORPHAN DISEASES

Most diseases involve only one organ system, such as the lungs or the heart. If treatment of a patient with, say, lung disease, is difficult to manage, patients are referred to a respirologist, an internist who specializes in diseases of the lung. If the internist cannot treat the lung disease with medications, then the patient may be referred to a thoracic surgeon, if the treatment requires surgery. But what happens if the cause of a condition is not within a single organ system? Who looks after those patients?

These are "orphan diseases" since no recognized group of physicians look after these problems. An example of an orphan disease is skin ulcers of the leg. The causes of skin ulcers in adults are many including venous, arterial, neuropathic[75], and pressure-related. Because of the complexity of ulcers, this is a poorly taught subject both in medical school and nursing school. As a result, even though skin ulcers affect one percent of the adult population, they are not well managed because of limited understanding by the average physician and nurse. Skin ulcers could be managed by dermatologists (since they occur on the skin), orthopedic surgeons (since they can

---

75   Neuropathy: Disease of nerves that may cause numbness or weakness.

occur close to the ankle), plastic surgeons (because they occur on the skin), or vascular surgeons (since they are frequently operating on the leg). In practice, dermatologists prefer treating other skin conditions, orthopedic surgeons are primarily interested in hip and knee problems, and plastic surgeons are more interested in reconstructive surgery in other areas of the body. With no other specialties being interested in these conditions, by default, all patients with leg wounds become the domain of vascular surgeons.

The other problem with chronic foot wounds is that their healing takes time. Early discharge with home care nurses to look after the wound can be a hit-or-miss affair with patients bouncing back to hospital because of poor or no home care nursing available in their communities. Medium and long-term care rehabilitation beds are similarly scarce, so the only remaining option is to keep these patients in acute care beds. At any one time there, may be as many as 20 percent of the vascular surgery inpatients having some type of lower extremity wound problem, from an ulcer, to gangrene involving a toe or the entire leg.

In 2013, I gave a Divisional presentation about the impact of the foot wound problems on our ward, and the resources required to look after them. With the help of Sandy Strandberg, our medical records decision support, I compared the length of stay (LOS) in patients who had a toe or foot wound problem with the LOS of patients with more serious problems, namely AAA or carotid artery disease:

VGH Cases and LOS
Jan 1, 2010 to Dec 31, 2011

Procedure	Cases	TLOS (d)	ALOS (d)
CEA	213		4.3
EVAR	139		6.2
Foot	35	1370	39.1
Toe	72	1914	26.6

Table 2. Comparison of LOS following different operations. CEA = carotid endarterectomy, EVAR = endovascular aneurysm repair, TLOS (d) = total length of stay in days, ALOS (d) = average length of stay in days.

From the table, it is apparent that the LOS of patients with a toe or foot wound stay in hospital considerably longer than AAA or carotid surgery patients. But, *four weeks* for a toe wound and almost *six weeks* for a foot wound! How could a simple problem like this occupy so much of the ward resources? These numbers are collected annually, and the figures are unchanged from year to year. We brought this to the attention of the hospital administration, but no potential solutions were recommended.

If necessity is the mother of invention, then when *do* we invent something to deal with this issue? Since surgery of chronic foot wounds is generally simple (debridement, toe amputation, skin grafting), we proposed transferring patients to the outpatient clinic to perform their minor foot surgery under local anesthetic. Our suggestions (which seemed so logical) were met with roadblocks. The responses we received ranged from: "There is no protocol," "What about patient transport," "We don't have the instruments," "What if the patients have MRSA," to: "What if the patients have a complication," etc. Funny how "No" can be said in so many different ways!

To handle these inpatient and outpatient foot problems and get patients either home sooner or have their care closer to home, the idea of a vascular centre was entertained: a place where an experienced nurse clinician could coordinate the inspection and treatment of these problems, and a place to serve as a teaching centre for medical students, residents, and nursing students. But in order to do this, we needed to fundraise.

20

FUNDRAISING AND AWARDS

The Peter Parker principle states that "with great power comes great responsibility." As physicians, let alone vascular surgeons, we have an immensely privileged role with respect to mentoring students and looking after patients. This role comes with great responsibility. Patients may wish to honour us (and our hospitals) with gifts. With the right financially successful patient, these gifts can be developed into endowments to support new or ongoing activities, or can be used for capital purchases. On the other hand, we may be the donor creating legacies of awards for talented or notable trainees to pursue further career choices. The UBC Vascular Surgery Division has had the good fortune of being able to do both.

Fundraising

We never started with a specific target or amount for fundraising. Rather, the money fell into our lap and beat us over the head, since we did not know what to do with it. The earliest example was an appreciative patient of Peter Fry's, who offered a six-figure donation for Peter and the division. Using his charm, Peter had the original amount matched by other donors, in order to purchase two duplex ultrasound machines for the division.

Similarly, Tony Salvian's patient, Bill Rogers, himself an engineer, created an endowment to fund vascular surgery research, The Robert C. and Patricia F. Rogers Endowment (see "The Vascular Fellowship").

Working in a publicly funded health care system, the budget is always close to the bone. With new technology comes the need for new capital purchases. As most of the hospital budget is already spoken for in employee salaries, there is hardly any money for new capital purchases, let alone new ideas to improve patient quality and safety or increase efficiency. Thus, each year there are a limited number of new capital projects that can be funded. If a project can be jointly funded with external donors there is a greater chance of these projects being successfully completed.

In the early 2000s, when endovascular surgery was taking off, we recognized the need to fundraise for a vascular centre to serve many purposes. First, we were going to need excellent imaging facilities to do high quality work in endovascular surgery. It was obvious that we were not welcome in other parts of the hospital such as Radiology or the Cardiac cath lab, so fund-raising efforts would need to be directed toward improvements in the OR. Second, vascular patients were becoming more complex as we struggled to keep patching them up in order to make a silk purse from a sow's ear. It would be ideal to have a dedicated location where the specialists we frequently interacted with, namely those from Cardiology, Neurology, and Nephrology, could be close at hand. Third, our ward was being overrun with foot wound problems (see "Orphan Diseases").

Of all the purposes for our fundraising efforts, the idea that caught the imagination of the donors was the largest piece of machinery:

a ceiling-mounted digital fluoroscope. After a multi-million-dollar purchase, and troubleshooting the software, it was installed in VGH OR #1 in 2017.

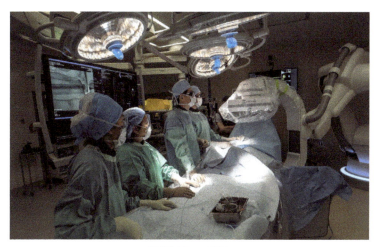

VGH OR. c. 2018.

Creating an Award

In 2007, I proposed an award for excellent junior general surgery residents to entice them to consider vascular surgery as a career. It would be a named award after one of the original surgeons and one of my mentors, Henry Hildebrand. In discussing the award, I had written to the other divisional members:

> "April 11, 2007
> Dear friends and colleagues,
> **RE: Dr. Henry D. Hildebrand Award**
>
> I would like to inform you of a new initiative to create a new award for junior general surgery residents, named in the honour of Dr. H. D. Hildebrand.

Over the past several years, I have been disappointed with the low number of applications and occasionally low quality of applicants to our Vascular Surgery training program. I can understand there may be many factors that contribute to this—age of resident, length of training, costs, lifestyle, and possibly gender issues, that dissuade many suitable applicants from applying. On the other hand, I believe that our specialty will be in high demand with the aging population and is particularly vibrant with the rapid development of endovascular surgery.

In particular, I am convinced that the UBC General Surgery training program produces outstanding residents, many of whom would make excellent vascular surgeons to serve BC and Canada in the future. I am a firm believer that, with a little more coaxing, we can encourage these fine young men and women to consider a career in vascular surgery.

Looking back on my own career, I had many mentors, including Dr. Henry Hildebrand. An outstanding clinical surgeon, Henry set very high standards for residents and fellows to emulate. Thus, it is fitting to create an award for General Surgery residents and encourage them to consider a career in Vascular Surgery, while honouring Henry at the same time.

This award will be $500…"

I was fully prepared to fund the award personally, but for once we got an overwhelming acceptance and agreement that the division would fund the award. The award was formally presented in 2009 with the first recipient being Andrea Rowe (now MacNeil), who ultimately chose a career in surgical oncology. The following year, Virginia Gunn was the winner. This time we achieved success as Virginia did transfer later to Vascular Surgery (see "End of the Fellowship and Birth of the Residency").

However, in 2012, the Royal College of Physicians and Surgeons of Canada created a direct entry program into vascular surgery. This meant that new residents would be selected from final year medical students and no longer needed to complete general surgery training prior to pursuing a subspecialty in vascular surgery. For the Hildebrand Award, it no longer made sense to continue in its current form with the stated purpose of attracting general surgery residents to vascular surgery. Thus, the Hildebrand Award was changed to medical students who wished to pursue vascular surgery, but even there it was difficult, as we had no control over what medical students wished to do in the future and what programs they would be matched to. The last winner of the award was Katie Duncan in 2014, who was matched to general surgery.

Although this may be the end of this award, there are so many excellent reasons for developing awards: from encouraging students to pursue vascular surgery, to "cross fertilization" of exchange students and residents, as well as to encourage excellence in clinical care and research. One just needs to have imagination and be able to recognize an opportunity.

If you don't do it, no one will. – Deryck Foster

21

What is a Surgeon's Time Worth?

If asked, "How much do you think a surgeon makes?" most lay people would estimate that their income is in the thousands or perhaps millions of dollars each year. Although that may apply to a few surgeons, such as plastic surgeons for the Hollywood stars, the reality is that in a publicly funded single payer system, surgeons are well paid, but nowhere like professional sports stars. An annual income in the hundreds of thousands is common but seven figures or more is almost unheard of.

These publicly available figures are the *gross* income, or the amount surgeons receive for medical services provided. Since surgeons, like most physicians, are small business owners, their business practice is fee-for-service, meaning they bill the provincial services plan within the Ministry of Health for medical services provided. As small business owners, they are responsible for the expenses of running a business, including rent, staff salaries, membership fees, etc. But the largest deduction from their annual salary is tax. In the end, the "take home" amount varies from 30–50 percent of the gross income.

For surgeons who work in academic centres, most income is still earned on a fee-for-service basis, but there are other responsibilities including teaching and research. The latter are not funded by the Ministry of Health, but through the Ministry of Education, whose budget for university educators is much less than that required to fund physicians. Although the mandates of academic health centres may be attractive for academically focused physicians, how do you incentivize physicians to do academic activities if they are far less well-compensated than when providing clinical service?

To examine this further, compare what a surgeon receives for clinical services with what they receive for teaching. In the clinic, the compensation for a vascular surgery consult is just over one hundred dollars; this amount is the same irrespective of how complicated the consult may be. In one hour, it is possible to see as many as four patients with the same simple problem, meaning the surgeon could earn as much as $400 per hour. On the other hand, if the problem is more complicated and the time required is thirty to forty-five minutes, then in one hour they could earn considerably less, perhaps $200 per hour. In the operating room, some operations are simpler than others; this is reflected in the billing amounts. For example, for a simple Hickman line procedure, which can be accomplished within twenty minutes, the compensation is around $300. But since the turnover time precludes doing two Hickman lines in an hour, the procedure is still worth $300 per hour. Other procedures that are far more complicated may pay up to $1200 for the procedure, but those procedures take four to five hours including turnover time. Plus, that amount includes everything from the pre-op planning to two weeks of post-op care. A Hickman line case usually requires no pre-op planning and involves no post-op care. So, multiple small cases can be as economically valuable as a large complicated case.

On the other hand, compensation provided to a clinical teacher for medical student teaching pays around one hundred dollars per hour. So, grossly, a surgeon can earn around $400 per hour looking after patients compared with one hundred dollars per hour for teaching.

For fee-for-service physicians, their income can be considerably affected with budgetary cutbacks. If a hospital's annual budget is reduced by the Ministry of Health, then one way of decreasing hospital costs without invoking the ire of labour unions is to decrease overall activities—this means bed and Operating Room (OR) closures so less labour is needed, fewer tests are performed, and fewer procedures are done. Although this is effective in holding the line on hospital expenditures, there are also profound consequences for (patients and) hospital physicians. Generally, most surgeons have only one to two days in the OR weekly to operate on patients. Since most surgeons' income is derived from operating, and not seeing patients in clinic, OR closures have a dramatic downward effect on surgeon incomes.

I experienced this first-hand on a number of occasions. Each OR day was about nine hours for scheduled, or elective, cases. After that, emergency cases that had been lined up that day, or from previous days, were undertaken. With reduced hospital budgets leading to reduced OR nursing staff, the ORs tightly controlled the elective cases by not letting cases run over their allotted time. Usually, the OR manager would patrol the rooms by one o'clock in the afternoon to see if cases were on schedule. If cases were running longer than planned, the upcoming elective cases would be cancelled. Unfortunately, due to the unpredictable nature of vascular surgery, some cases would take longer than others. It should be recognized that the surgeon's focus is always on the patient immediately in front of them, and not the next case. Nonetheless, it did not matter what the reason was for a case to run late—whether due to a late start by the anesthetist, a slow turnover time, or anything else, it always became the surgeon's responsibility.

This would take its toll on teaching in the OR as well. If the case was potentially late, the surgeon would take the reins to get through it on time. And if the case was truly late and the next case was cancelled, then the surgeon's responsibility was to personally inform their next patient that their surgery was cancelled and would need to be rebooked. OR rooms were allowed to remain empty rather than trying to fit in the final case and risk letting it run over, even for an hour or less. Then, to rub salt in the wound, everybody from the cleaners to nurses would be paid except for the surgeon, since their reimbursement was fee-for-service.

The continued ups and downs of budgetary restrictions had further effects, not only on clinical incomes, but also on retaining surgeons and recruiting new ones. But what would be a fair process to compensate surgeons in academic centres? Examining gross incomes alone, there were large variations. Even though the hospital resources, including beds, call schedules, and OR time were equally divided, larger incomes equated to those who were working and billing more. Higher billing surgeons may have been more efficient in seeing more patients in their clinics or they were working longer hours. For those with lower gross incomes, they may have been less efficient or were doing more activities that paid less, such as teaching and research.

Despite the variation in gross billing, there was a desire to achieve a more equitable funding arrangement that would recognize the roles of a surgeon in an academic institution. Enter the concept of "practice plans." These were a socialist-style model of more equitable compensation for all members of a group such as a department-wide practice plan. Originally implemented in parts of Eastern Canada, practice plans combined the gross clinical incomes and academic stipends of all members, and redistributed funds to individual surgeons based on their clinical contributions and academic productivity. At VGH and UBC, lacking the leadership for a department-wide plan, most divisions negotiated with the Ministry of Health through their hospitals.

After several attempts, the VGH Division of Vascular Surgery negotiated a clinical service contract with the hospital in 2011. This contract was for clinical services only. Academic activities continued with compensation from the university being based on the number of hours spent teaching. Other divisions negotiated their own contracts; some were a clinical academic service contract, meaning there were academic expectations, but most were clinical service contracts.

The transition from a fee-for-service model to a clinical services contract was met with enthusiasm as it meant that one's income was stable irrespective of the ups and downs of hospital slowdowns, out of town meetings, or vacations, which, under the fee-for-service model, were never compensated. I valued the extra freedom, spending more time with patients by explaining their problems, options, risks, and benefits more thoroughly. To me, being on a clinical service contract meant I could become a much better physician. I also became a far better teacher in the OR. Unshackled from the risk of cancelled surgeries, I reduced my OR bookings to allow residents more time to do operations under supervision.

However, it also created unexpected behaviour. Under the old fee-for-service model, surgeons diligently examined rosters to ensure equitable resources. Vacations were taken sparingly knowing that time away meant that there was no income for those periods. With service contracts, "shadow billing"[76] was required as a means of tracking clinical productivity to ensure it would not drop off precipitously. Vacation time was now carefully watched as everybody took all of their allotted time off; nobody wanted to be working any more than they needed to.

Everything considered, having a clinical service contract was a welcome boon for the program. It removed any jealousies around income disparity, allowed physicians to pursue clinical and teaching excellence, and allowed greater subspecialization. The need to shadow bill (with the potential threat of cancelling the contract) is always present, but after years of medical school and residency training, surgeons have been trained to be obsessive and compulsive individuals who enjoy working hard.

76   Shadow billing: fee for service billing continues (to a third party) even with a service contract that provides a regular salary. It provides a guide to determine if productivity remains the same.

22

End of the Fellowship and Birth of the Residency (2012)

Toward the end of the first decade of the 2000s, there was a growing recognition of the need to change the traditional "5+2" (five years of general surgery residency and two years of vascular fellowship) paradigm of vascular surgery training. With the endovascular revolution sweeping across all vascular units, numerous new skills would need to be taught. General surgery training was also becoming less relevant to the practice of vascular surgery, as most of the abdominal general surgical procedures were endoscopic cases. In addition, this model was limited to recruiting only those graduating general surgeons who still had fire in the belly after medical school and general surgery residency. With older medical students, more female medical students, and residents now graduating with more debt than ever before, the quality and quantity of applicants seeking additional training in vascular surgery was falling.

We could see it with the progressively fewer applicants to our fellowship program. For some years, there would only be one or two applicants. In those lean years, the major decision amongst the staff was whether we would go without a fellow and make do with other surgical residents for call coverage and intraoperative assistance, or take whatever candidate was available. However, there was concern that not taking a fellow and not using the available funding from the postgraduate office could lead to not getting funding for future fellows. As a result, we invariably accepted all fellows, occasionally with some regret.

On a practical level, after five years of general surgery most new vascular fellows were good at things that were not useful to vascular surgery, such as endoscopic skills, and few had senior resident skills that were useful to vascular surgery, namely dissecting out blood vessels, and sewing. We had seen that all of the first-year general surgery residents could easily become proficient in basic vascular surgical skills by the end of a two-month rotation. However, after that first rotation, their open surgical skills were not developed further as they returned to their programs and focused on laparoscopic surgery. It seemed that the only additional exposure to sewing blood vessels came during a rotation in hepatobiliary surgery and liver transplantation.

As a result, the first year of the two-year vascular fellowship was often spent undoing bad habits acquired during general surgery training and reteaching the basics to produce proficient and efficient technicians.

And now they needed to learn endovascular techniques. For traditional open surgery, after deciding who needs an operation, the mindset is linear, starting from the incision (where, how large) to the middle and frequently critical part of the procedure, and finally to the closure and denouement. Along the way, key traps to avoid falling into "What would you do if you fell into that trap?" are rehearsed in private by the surgeon and aloud with the students and residents. Others would recognize this as the formulation of a "plan B" if "plan A" goes sideways.

Endovascular is entirely different. The approach is not from the outside to inside, as in traditional surgery peeling back the onion layers, but instead, an inside-out approach. In order to get to where you want to be, you need access. Access to the circulation initially, then access to the lesion in question. If location, location, location, is the mantra of real estate, then access, access, access, is the mantra of endovascular. Along the way, it requires the right tools. First, a guide (wire) platform over which all other devices can pass. A new vocabulary must be learned for all the different wires, catheters, and devices. Each have specific names and sizes, but share one thing in common—each device only does one thing, owing to its size or shape. So it becomes necessary to change devices because of anatomy (sometimes tortuous, sometimes progressively smaller) to get to where you want to be. Then you need to need to know what devices fit into what, much like a trombone. As a result, for the planning of an endovascular procedure, the planning is backwards from the final device to what can carry it there, the necessary catheters or guidewires required, until finally what initial device (sheath) will be needed for the initial access to the circulation.

The Americans recognized this need earlier, and by the late 2000s were offering a vascular integrated residency: a five-year program post medical school instead of, or sometimes in parallel with, the traditional 5+2 vascular fellowship program. The Royal College of Physicians and Surgeons of Canada also created a five-year direct entry residency program into vascular surgery (see "Fundraising and Awards"). Its inaugural year was 2012, and all ten sites across the country rolled this out to replace the vascular fellowship program, except for the University of Toronto, which maintained a dual fellowship and residency program.

For the first year of this new program, we were allowed to "poach" junior residents from general surgery and select a direct entry medical student. In our first year, we recruited Sandra Jenneson and Virginia Gunn from General Surgery. It turned out Sandra had always wanted a career in emergency medicine and within two months she left for the emergency medicine program. Virginia, who had always wanted to pursue a career in vascular surgery, continued and graduated as our first resident graduate in 2015. Our first direct entry medical student was Jon Misskey. Jon was an exceptional resident and pursued a master's in health profession education during the residency. Jon graduated in 2019 and was appointed as staff at VGH the same year.

Being able to train residents at an early stage has allowed rapid assimilation of both endovascular and open surgical training. Unlike the long period of dormancy for vascular fellows, in the residency program surgical skills have improved with more frequent and progressively challenging surgical procedures. Concerns about not having adequate open operative experience for aortic surgery or abdominal pathology have proved to be overblown. Our centre still does a large number of open aortic and peripheral limb bypasses, which makes it conducive to training well rounded surgeons.

The King is dead. Long live the King.

23

BC Vascular (Surgery) Day
(2014 – 2018)

Unlike in the US, the creation of staff or consultant positions for Canadian hospital-based physicians is a constant struggle, since government funding determines the number of available hospital positions. This occurs irrespective of the population number, age mix, or development of new diseases. For a specialty like surgery, this is particularly acute, since all surgeons need to work in hospitals.

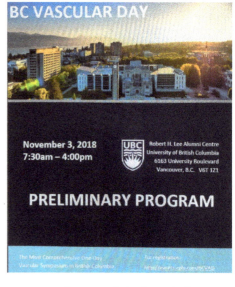

For vascular surgery, this is no different. In 2014, as I heard the anguish about the lack of job prospects from our then senior resident, Virginia Gunn, I decided to create the BC Vascular Surgery Day. The problem, I surmised, was not that the residents were not getting good training, but that they were not known in BC, where most of them hoped to find employment.

The primary purpose of BC Vascular Surgery Day was to create a forum whereby the residents could be introduced to their potential future partners, the vascular surgeons of BC. We developed a program that featured each resident either presenting a case or discussing a topic. In addition, we allowed ample time for mingling afterwards.

Featured speakers were considered. Our loose criteria were that they should be an accomplished UBC alumnus or a well-known vascular surgeon who would be able to give an inspiring talk. Dr. Jack Pacey, a general and vascular surgeon based at Burnaby General Hospital, was selected to be the inaugural speaker. Jack had been immensely successful as a surgeon and an inventor and agreed to talk on "Developing Clinical Ideas into Business Ventures."

The first meeting was held at the Hotel Georgia in downtown Vancouver, and funding was provided by the many device companies. Everything was set, except for the surgeons. I should have known this. Many years earlier, as the last president of the Westcoast Vascular Society, we had to dissolve that small society after 1995 because of poor attendance.

For this event, every BC vascular surgeon had been contacted, and to entice them to attend, we planned an economic forum during the BC Vascular Surgery Day, to discuss billing issues. This brought out a few from Victoria, New Westminster, and Kelowna, but it was nowhere near the overwhelming response I had hoped for.

With only a handful of attending surgeons and the residents, how could we salvage the day with around forty empty seats? After some consideration, I made the decision to proceed based on the recognition that a successful meeting requires bums in seats. So we filled the seats with nurses from the ward, as well as from the OR.

Now with a packed house, and also allowing the company reps to give a brief talk on updates from each company, the day was off to a roaring start. It was more than we had hoped for, except for the original purpose—residents still did not get the opportunity to meet their potential future partners. On top of that, the economic forum was a closed-door meeting excluding the residents, something that made no sense at the time, and still doesn't.

The following two years were the same format, with Dr. Gerrit Winkelaar, and then Dr. David Kopriva, being the keynote speakers. However, this was becoming more of a nursing education meeting and an opportunity for industry to show their wares. During the third BCVSD, one of the mid-level residents, Gary Yang, asked what the residents could do *in lieu* of being banished from the economic forum.

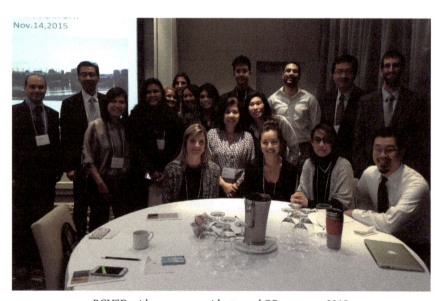

BCVSD with surgeons, residents, and OR nurses. c. 2015.

For the next two years, recognizing that growth was needed in view of the success of the meeting, the venue was changed to the new UBC Alumni Centre. Dr. Jim Dooner was the keynote speaker. In addition, when the economic forum was happening in the afternoon, the residents would organize their own afternoon workshops directed to family physicians and family practice residents. If they were not allowed to attend the economic forum, then a more direct sale approach to the family practitioners might be beneficial for their future practice. This format was a tremendous success, but required a significant amount of work and organization.

The final BCVSD in 2018 was renamed the BC Vascular Day (BCVAD) to recognize the myriad of other specialists that attended as speakers. The meeting had both educational and entertainment value, with a debate and Jeopardy session for the audience. Dr. Husain Khambati was the featured speaker. The afternoon sessions now included rehab medicine, sports cardiology (at UBCH), cardiac surgery, ward nursing, OR nursing, as well as the resident-run practical sessions on ultrasound, stent grafts, angioplasty, and stents for family physicians and family practice residents.

That was the last BCVSD or BCVAD. It had outgrown its original intent and become a forum for cardiovascular care. It was a useful community event, but now that it had strayed so far from its primary purpose, I was no longer interested in organizing it. The formula is still there for anybody willing to take up the torch, but unfortunately, we did not create any succession planning for others to take over.

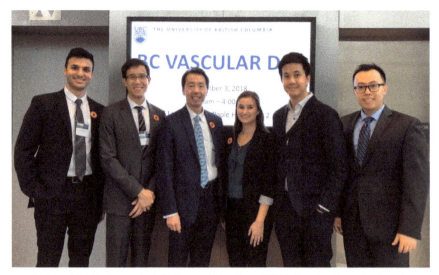

Left to right. Residents Abdalla Butt, Adrian Fung, YNH, Eva Angelopoulos (admin assistant), Gary Yang, Bill Huang. c. 2018.

Predicting human behaviour is near impossible. Whatever you think may happen usually does not. But, if the behaviour turns into something favourable, you should go with it. Organizing this event has reinforced the notion that while many people talk about doing things (that may lead to change), there are very few who will actually attempt to do it.

24

Development of the Vascular Engineering Research Group (VERG)

For those of us who have wished to go back in time when things were simpler, the opportunity arose for me in 2011. By then, I had relinquished most of my administrative responsibilities, and was concentrating on clinical care, teaching, and research.

Clinical care is extremely rewarding, having the privilege of entering a patient's private world of disease, deciding and executing a plan, and seeing the patient through their path. Most surgical patients, though, need to go through some degree of pain and suffering before they get better. Even though their lives may be improved, many would not want to go through the same experience again.

Teaching is similarly rewarding by observing the growth of students and residents when they finally grasp a concept or achieve a technical goal. It's the equivalent of watching your flower bloom after a prolonged period of toil and sweat.

Unlike clinical care and teaching, which only improves the situation for one person or a handful, research has the ability to affect hundreds to thousands of patients. However, *high quality* research is the most challenging of all those activities. Being a successful researcher requires many things that are not required in the practice of medicine or teaching. In addition to specific training, it requires curiosity, innovation, and stubbornness. The latter is the most important quality since the number of roadblocks to high quality research is immense. From unfunded grant applications (the successful funding rate is about 10 percent of applications), to abstract and paper submissions and rejections, to delays in everything from factors such as ethics review to labour action, the list of hurdles for a successful researcher to overcome is long.

In addition, nobody can know everything, which means that a researcher will require research partners. The life of a researcher is actually not much different than that of a person working in another specialized discipline, such as business. Although you have expertise in your area, your expertise is limited, and you need to bring in specialists who can add to your idea or enhance your theories. These specialists, now your associates or co-principal investigators (co-PI), can enhance your group's overall expertise, but may also introduce unexpected personal dynamics.

I learned two truths very early on regarding co-investigators: you can't live without them, and you can't kill them (to borrow from a famous quote). When deciding on a partnership, do you choose the most experienced person who may have the worst personality, or do you work with someone less competent, but with whom you can get along? Often life's problems can be summarized in graphs. When choosing a co-investigator based on competence and personality, the choices can be summarized in the following graph:

COMPETENCE VS. PERSONALITY

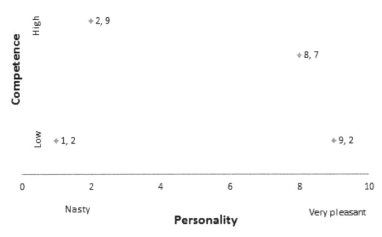

Table 3. Comparison of personality and competence.

Ideally, we would want somebody who is extremely competent and has an excellent personality, so that appears in the upper right-hand corner of the chart. On the other hand, the person to avoid is the minimally competent person with a nasty personality, or the lower left-hand corner. In between, though, is the tough decision of working with somebody competent with a less desirable personality or somebody not very competent, but simply a nice person. The usual dilemma is between these choices.

Having worked with co-investigators of all types, my early experience was working with co-investigators found in the upper left-hand corner, namely those who were extremely good at what they did, but I would later discover a dark side to their personalities. Short-term, but no long-term, success was achieved since the thought of working with them in another long-term project was horrendous.

Later reflection allows you to wonder: "What if I had worked with that nice person, even though they are not the most talented?"

In 2011, I was at a point in my career where I could be reflective. And on reflection, the most satisfying part of my research career was working collaboratively with the engineers. The cross fertilization of fluid dynamic concepts with human biology was stimulating for all of us, and thinking about how improving the available knowledge through research could benefit many thousands of patients was an elixir we all drank from.

I contacted Sheldon Green, my counterpart in 1992, to check his availability to restart a new Engineering-Vascular Surgery collaboration. Sheldon was now the department head of Mechanical Engineering, and inundated with administration, teaching, and his own research. He politely declined, but recommended a group of younger engineering professors to meet with me. Thus began my second partnership with Engineering.

Unlike my first experience, this new group of mechanical and electrical engineers had some knowledge of blood vessels and their diseases. The vascular surgeons' main contribution was showing them the clinical relevance of their discoveries and pointing out the areas where we needed their help in answering our clinical questions.

This alliance, including Joel Gagnon and me, along with mechanical engineer Srikanth Phani, electrical engineers Ken Takahata and Shahriar Mirabbasi, and our biomaterials expert, Jay Kizzakkedathu, was loosely known as the Vascular Engineering Research Group, or VERG.

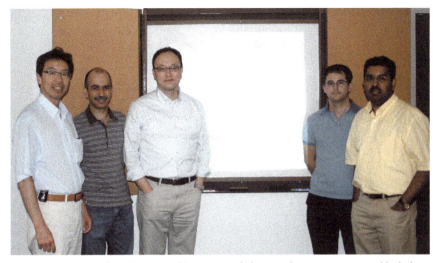

Left to Right: Myself, Shahriar Mirabbasi, Ken Takahata, Joel Gagnon, Jay Kizzakkedathu.
c. 2012.

This combination was deadly as our group was rewarded with four NSERC-CIHR grants in our first five attempts. We had novel ideas, from developing devices that could wirelessly detect intraluminal pressure changes (the publication made the cover of *Advanced Science*) (Chen et al 2018), and wirelessly heating stents to inhibit intimal hyperplasia[77] (Yi et al. 2019), to bendable catheters that could negotiate changing vascular anatomy, to novel blood vessel and organ sealants for blood conservation.

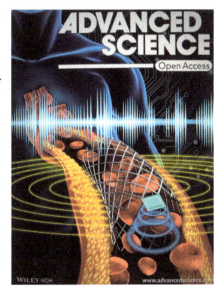

---

77   Intimal hyperplasia: a pathological process of wound healing that leads to re-narrowing of blood vessels following treatment.

This was the new model to advance vascular research: bold new ideas that arose from knowledge of disease and the application of new technology to treat our nemeses.

PART FIVE

THE VGH
VASCULAR SURGEONS

From 1978 to 2020 there have been thirteen past and present staff surgeons in the VGH Division of Vascular Surgery. Despite their different backgrounds, all received their vascular surgery training at UBC. Critics may decry this apparent inbreeding, but the varied backgrounds did show through in their style of practice, teaching approaches, and pursuit of higher knowledge through research. The long observational period during fellowship or residency allowed the surgeons to deliberately choose not only new surgeons with ability, but also personalities that would be compatible with the group. The following is a glimpse into their backstories.

Dr. Wallace Bakfu Chung, MD CM, FRCSC, FACS, DSc (Hon.), OBC, OC

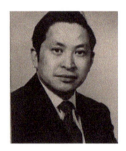

Successful physician, surgeon, administrator, educator, and donor, Dr. Wally Chung has a special place in many people's hearts. His fascinating life story has one rarely publicized example of quick thinking and organizational skills. Born into a large Chinese Canadian family in Victoria, BC, Wally was the first son to attend university and successfully enter McGill University Medical School. Upon graduation, Wally returned to VGH for internship.

As an intern, he spent a one-month rotation at Pearson Hospital, then the site treating many long-term rehabilitation patients, including patients with poliomyelitis that affected their diaphragms. These patients had no muscle control over their diaphragms and other muscles of respiration. In order to assist their breathing, they were kept in iron lung machines: negative pressure mechanical respirators which enables patients to breathe on their own.

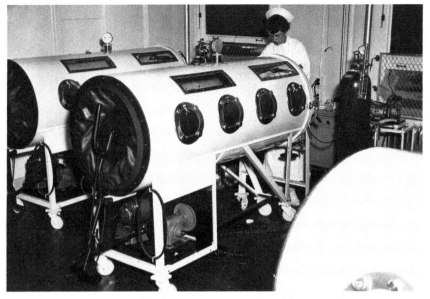

Iron Lung. (Credit: Vancouver Coastal Health 1.1/742a)

Bored, Wally spent time around the iron lung machines, inquiring about the knobs and levers that would ventilate the patient should there be an electrical failure.

As the number of polio patients who needed mechanical ventilation increased, Pearson Hospital continued to add more patients in iron lungs to their hospital.

In 1953, as the intern stationed at Pearson, Wally had to act fast when the fuse box failed, leaving the large open ward in complete darkness. With no more hissing from the iron lungs, Wally knew that patients would soon be dying—fast. If every cloud has a silver lining, then this cloud's lining was that the fuse box exploded at afternoon shift change. The morning shift's nurses and orderlies had not yet left, and the afternoon staff were just arriving. Wally quickly gathered all the nurses and orderlies to inform them of the situation and instigated a plan to keep the patients alive until the fuse box could be repaired.

Each iron lung has a mechanical lever at the foot of the cylindrical container for just such occasions. The combined staff were ordered to arrange every two iron lungs with their foot ends facing each other so one person could grasp the levers from each cylinder and mechanically ventilate two iron lungs simultaneously. Regardless of nurse or orderly, each would continue to do this until fatigued, then another staff person would take over the levering duties. The rate of levering would be dependent on the patient—their level of consciousness, and whether they were becoming cyanotic or not.

This went on for at least an hour, no doubt an eternity for the staff and patients alike, until the fuse box was fixed. Wally's heroic action that day saved the life of every iron lung patient.

The next day, Wally and the staff were summoned into the superintendent's office. Expecting to be praised, or at least offered a nice lunch for their efforts, Wally and the staff, to their surprise, found the superintendent's office filled with lawyers. Instead of being praised for their quick thinking and professionalism, they were told, in no uncertain terms, never to mention this incident to anyone. It was to have never existed. No newspapers or reporters were informed of the true story of that afternoon at Pearson Hospital.

Dejected, Wally left the room confused and went back to his life as a lowly intern. With that episode behind him, he continued to work hard and was accepted into progressive professional and leadership roles: surgery resident, chief resident, attending staff, division and department head, and professor of surgery.

Years later at a hospital function, Wally saw the Pearson superintendent again. After exchanging pleasantries, the superintendent asked Wally about his career. When Wally told him that life had been kind and he had the good fortune of receiving every promotion he applied for, the superintendent seemed to be very pleased. "Remember the Pearson Hospital incident in 1953?" he asked. "At the time, we couldn't mention anything that would show your heroism and our incompetence, but we had to thank you somehow." And, in this way, he contributed to the legacy of Wally Chung.

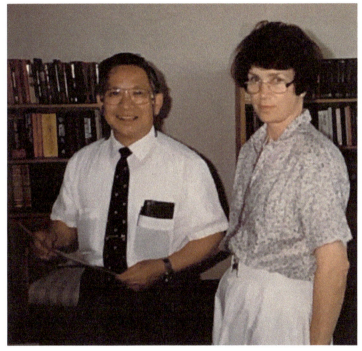

Wally Chung and Madelaine Bicknell (Surgery Administrator) c. 1978.

"Success occurs when opportunity meets preparation." – Zig Ziglar

Dr. Henry Knowles Litherland, MA, MB BCh, FRCSC

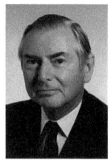

Dr. Henry Litherland was born in Wigan, England into a medical family. Growing up during World War II, Henry joined the Royal Air Force (RAF) at age seventeen after completing high school. After proudly serving for six years as a fighter pilot in Palestine and Cyprus, flying Spitfires and Vampire jets, he retired from the RAF in 1953 and returned to Cambridge University to pursue medical training.

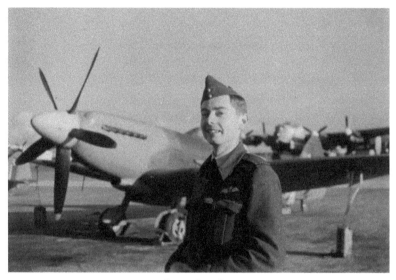

HKL in front of Spitfire. c. 1948.

In his memoir (generously provided by sons Peter and Simon Litherland), he details life in mid-century England as a medical student, then house officer: studying and being on the wards, rowing with the Cambridge team, living the life of characters in the *Doctor in the House* series, and many European jaunts in his trusted MG packed with boats.

After his house officer years, Henry, along with a number of expatriate English physicians, decided to leave the UK, as they had no faith in the National Health Service (NHS). As his younger brother, Oswald, was already living in Canada, Henry wished to be closer to him and applied for higher training as a surgical resident at the Veterans' Hospital in Victoria, BC in 1961. After one year in Victoria, he was accepted as an associate resident, initially in pathology, at VGH before transferring to general surgery. Henry completed his general surgery training in 1965 and started his career in general and vascular surgery at VGH in 1966 (Litherland, H. Unpublished).

When the new Vascular Surgery Division was created by Wally Chung, Henry was invited to become one of its members. Henry's academic career took off from there; he became the head of Vascular Surgery in 1986 and associate head of Surgery in 1990. Henry had also developed a passion for computers and became the director for Computing Services for the Department of Surgery in 1977. His passion for computers continued at home, but in order to appease his wife, Audrey, with his new toy, he first needed to buy her a diamond ring.

His surgical skill even extended to animals. Two incidents involving cats were fondly recalled by his son, Simon: ". . . he also took the stitches out of the cat when it got an infection. The vet was not happy because cats heal differently than people. There was an earlier cat that had a kidney problem and the vet (the same one) said to Mom, 'Bring him back tomorrow after you tell the family and I'll put him down.' Anyhow, Dad had some drugs from experimental kidney transplants which he was doing at the time—I think he gave Morris some cyclosporine which seemed to do the trick as the cat lived another five years and died at twenty-two. I think that's when Dad has been the saddest: he was always in bad shape when patients died and when our cats and dogs died, even when he knew that he had done his best."

Henry passed away in late November 2012. Although he had passed away earlier, Henry Hildebrand's description of Henry Litherland summed up perfectly his colleague and friend:

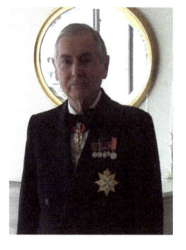

"Nobody could have wished for a better partner. Henry Litherland was a typical English gentleman with integrity, generosity, understanding, and tolerance of my shortcomings. In the thirty years we worked together we never once had a major disagreement."

For an Englishman, could there be any greater accomplishment than being an RAF pilot and a vascular surgeon?

Dr. Henry Daniel Hildebrand, MD, FRCSC

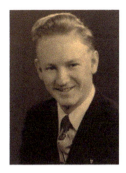

Dr. Henry Hildebrand was born into a large Mennonite family in rural southern Manitoba. His parents were poor farmers and struggled to make ends meet. Along with his parents and eleven siblings, Henry lived in a small shack ("the rat house," he called it). Despite the austere conditions, Henry found enjoyment with simple things to while away the time. He was a mischievous young lad who, with religion and determination, became the first member of his family to graduate in medicine.

Working as a CPR porter, he travelled with the train frequently to Vancouver, a city on the move to young Henry, and where he wished to one day live.

His dream to live in Vancouver did not come true until he finished his years as a missionary physician. In 1958, Henry took his young family to the Belgian Congo, expecting to work for four years. After two years, they had to evacuate promptly due to the Congo's sudden independence movement and forthcoming civil war (Hildebrand HK 2006).

Upon returning to Canada, he worked for eighteen months as a general practitioner, long enough to realize that he preferred being a surgeon. He applied and was accepted as a surgery resident at Shaughnessy Hospital in Vancouver for one year before completing his general surgery residency at VGH. He started his career in general surgery at VGH in 1966, and shared an office with Henry Litherland for the next thirty years. After doing both general and vascular surgery, in 1981 he tailored his practice to only vascular surgery.

Henry had excellent oratorical skills and with his devotion to religion, he was a regular speaker at the Killarney Park Mennonite Brethren Church, as well as serving on the board of governors of Regent College for fourteen years. When he retired from practice in 1996, he answered a calling to return to Africa and worked for six months at the Africa Inland Mission Hospital in Kijabe, Kenya (Hildebrand HD 2006).

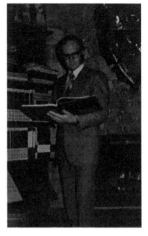

Henry carried the mischievous streak he was born with throughout his life, though sometimes it seemed that hilarious events followed him wherever he went. In his autobiography, Henry recalls the time he saw a patient in the ER with an ischemic foot from a femoral artery occlusion. Paradoxically, the foot was beet red instead of being as white as a sheet. Knowing that occasionally patients with acute gout may have a similar presentation, Henry asked the man if he ever had gout. With a thick Eastern European accent, the man declared: "I've had a sheep and a pig but never a goat!" (*ibid.*)

This mischievous trait was also passed on to his children. While his oldest son, Lloyd, was driving the family across the country in their 1962 Mercury, Henry awoke from his slumber to discover the scenery passing by at an alarming rate. When he asked, "What the hell are you doing?" to Lloyd, his son shot back an approving look and proudly announced, "Oh, around ninety!"

But sometimes Henry got comments as good as he could dish out. In the 1980s and 1990s, political correctness was not even on anyone's radar. Henry enjoyed teasing the students and had his standard question about the hypoglossal nerve whenever there was a female student scrubbed in a carotid case. Henry would ask, "I am working in this part of the neck where there is an anatomic structure that is always larger in a female than a male. What is it?" But Henry finally met his match when a particularly astute female student said after reflection, "Oh, I know. It's the brain!" And with that, Henry never asked that question again (Hsiang 2020).

A master technician, he would always make everything look easy. He needled us, too, with sarcastic remarks about the rust that had accumulated on our instruments while he was out of the room. Or, maybe, he could make a surgeon out of us after 10,000 years!

His talents even extended to the weather, or at least to the seasons. Being ever the snappy dresser, Lynn Doyle always knew that spring had arrived when Henry turned up in his white patent leather shoes.

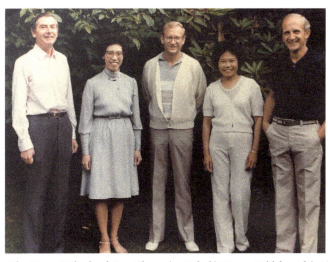

Left to right: Henry Litherland, Roz Chung (unit clerk), Henry Hildebrand (with white leather shoes), Letty Davidson (Head Nurse), Peter Fry. c. 1987.

After joining the VGH staff in 1994, I continued to work with Henry, but now as a surgical colleague. On October 3, 1995 both of us were working together in OR #4 when the announcement came in: O.J. was acquitted! It was as astonishing to us then as now. I can recall being in the room, but have no recollection of what the case was.

Unfortunately, Henry had a terrible family history of coronary artery disease. Although he managed to outlive his father and other male siblings, Henry required coronary angioplasty twice, as well as coronary artery bypass surgery. His experience with the latter was not pleasant. Waking up, he discovered an enormous hematoma from the saphenous vein harvest site. He admonished the cardiac resident with: "Do you know how long I have been doing this operation and never seen a hematoma this size?!" Even from home, he could not resist a dig at the nurses by calling the ward and saying in a hushed voice, "This is Dr. Hildebrand calling from heaven," or ". . . the rumours about my death are patently untrue." Those phone calls freaked out the nurses.

Humour aside, Henry could not outrun heart disease and died several heart beats from Valentine's Day, on February 13, 2008, aged 76. The notice of his passing that appeared in the Canadian Medical Association Journal included a segment of my eulogy: "He had so many fine qualities for a young resident like me to emulate. His surgical skill was peerless. A rare surgical athlete, he possessed speed, precision, and deftness of touch. He was the conductor in the operating room and all eyes were on his movements and subtle gestures" (CMAJ 2008).

Despite all of his surgical achievements, it was his compassion for his fellow man and for Africa that prompted him to establish the vesicovaginal fistula[78] fund through the African Inland Mission. This is the legacy he has left for us.

---

78   Vesicovaginal fistula: an abnormal connection between the bladder and vagina as a result of prolonged childbirth.

Dr. Peter Douglas Fry, FRCSI, FRCSC

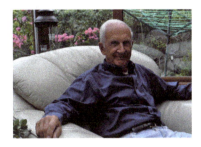

Dr. Peter Fry was born in the south of England and received his medical training at the Royal College of Surgeons of England. After completing the first part of his surgical training and not wanting to continue in the NHS, he applied to multiple institutions for higher training, choosing to complete his general surgery training in Vancouver. As a fourth-year surgery resident, Peter was influenced by Wally Chung to consider vascular surgery as a subspecialty. During this time, he visited Dr. Eugene Strandness in Seattle who impressed upon him the key role of ultrasound in the diagnosis of vascular disease.

After completing both Irish and Canadian fellowships in General Surgery, he worked with a cardiac surgeon, Dr. Robert Miyagishima, at SPH on liver disease, especially arterializing the portal venous system. After tragedy struck Tony Chan's family (see "Origins"), Peter was recruited by Wally to work at VGH. When UBCH opened in 1980, Peter joined Wally there while maintaining his obligations at VGH. It was at UBCH that Peter found his pioneering spirit in endovascular surgery.

Strongly influenced by Ted Dietrich, Peter sought to advance vascular surgery in non-invasive testing and introduce new less invasive techniques. In his presidential address to the Canadian

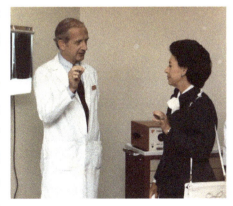

Explaining vascular surgery to HRH Princess Margaret. c. 1988.

Society for Vascular Surgery (CSVS) in 1989, Peter recommended that CSVS members take a more active role in developing new ideas and techniques while being wary of extravagant claims of success (Fry 1991). His concern was that if CSVS members did not take an active interest in these new developments, it would "deny those following." True to his word, he was the first surgeon in Canada to perform an argon-beam laser assisted balloon angioplasty[79] and the first endovascular aneurysm repair (EVAR).

As an educator, Peter influenced many trainees, including those from distant places such as the UK, the Middle East, and the Far East. All his residents learned about the way he could "make the needle dance on the graft," a technique of positioning the needle on the needle driver by balancing the tip of the needle on the graft while altering the location where the needle driver would clasp onto the needle.

In private life, Peter developed a passion for farming and bought a hobby farm in Langley, BC. Many of the farming tips he learned were from Henry Hildebrand. At the time he was working at UBCH, Peter would routinely wake up at an ungodly hour to commute from Langley, just to beat the residents rounding at seven o'clock in the morning. And, after a full day of surgery, he would make the return commute, sometimes to bale hay until midnight. Peter's favourite comment to anybody questioning his demanding schedule was, "You can get plenty of sleep once you're dead."

Peter retired from practice in 2018 and continues to live in Langley. He may have traded haying for weed whacking, but his work is never done.

---

79   Argon-beam laser assisted balloon angioplasty: balloon angioplasty supplemented with laser energy to create a working channel for a guidewire that allows a track for the balloon catheter to pass over.

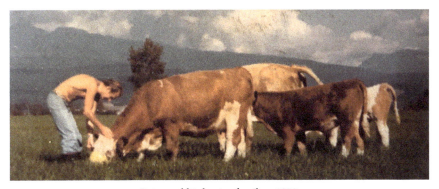

Peter and his bovine family. c.1978.

Dr. Anthony (Tony) John Salvian, MD, FRCSC

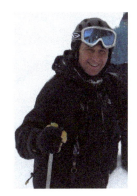

Dr. Tony Salvian was raised in Ontario where he went to medical school at the University of Western Ontario. Being part of the Baby Boomer generation, his favourite artist was Elvis Presley, and his favourite song was likely "Jailhouse Rock."

In 1976 he came west to Vancouver to complete a residency in general surgery. Stimulated by working with the VGH vascular surgeons, he did extra training in vascular surgery at the University of Manitoba under the guidance of Dr. Allan Downs, and then a brief fellowship with Dr. Wes Moore at UCLA.

Tony has always been a clinically focused surgeon, and from Winnipeg he brought back three new concepts. The first was using a two-suture technique for the anastomosis. Each suture was anchored at the heel and toe of the anastomosis. This would allow for improved visualization of the placement of sutures at the apices, with the resultant knots being tied in the middle of the anastomosis. Prior to this new technique, the fellows were taught to use a quicker (and "nastier") method of dividing a double-armed suture and anchoring the heel and toe of the anastomosis with a single half of the Prolene suture. This was definitely quicker, but the placement of the bites was invariably blind at the ends. The superior technique that Tony introduced was rapidly adopted.

The second technique was using a patch graft whenever a vertical arteriotomy was made.[80] This was absolutely necessary if the incision was made in a small artery and also preferably in a large artery as well. Patch graft closure (always autogenous with Tony) became routine following carotid endarterectomy. Prior to that, the carotid artery was closed primarily following endarterectomy by taking multiple small bites of the carotid artery. With routine ultrasound surveillance, any increased flow velocities due to small areas of narrowing or turbulence following primary closure were eliminated with patching.

The third technique he brought back was the "Winnipeg abdominal closure." This was a two layered closure for midline laparotomy incisions. There was the initial placement of interrupted non-absorbable Tevdek sutures, followed by a continuous non-absorbable suture (could be Prolene or PDS). Once the continuous suture layer was completed, the Tevdek sutures would be tied. Prior to this, the other surgeons were closing their laparotomy incisions with a single layer of continuous Dexon (an absorbable suture). However, the post-procedure ventral hernia rate was very high—up to 50 percent! Using the Winnipeg technique, the ventral hernia rate was much lower, less than 10 percent.

---

80   With a vertical incision, simply sewing it up may gather the surrounding tissue and cause narrowing. By sewing another piece of material into the closure site, this widens the space and reduces the risk of narrowing.

As Tony's focus was to provide exemplary vascular care to his patients, he became the main person for many problems, such as vascular access (see "Hickman Lines - The Second Skirmish with Radiology") and thoracic outlet syndrome. We were all grateful that Tony had such a dedicated interest in the management of thoracic outlet[81] issues. As a result, he became the local expert on thoracic outlet issues after soft tissue neck injuries following motor vehicle injuries. During the 1990s, and even now, the standard way of treating Paget-Schroetter disease[82] is venous thrombolysis[83] and first rib resection during the same admission. Tony was much more thoughtful, and believed that not all patients needed to have their first rib removed. He favoured a conservative "wait and see" approach and recommended rib resection only for those patients who remained symptomatic with persistent evidence of continued rib compression of their subclavian veins. This conservative approach was published in the *Journal of Vascular Surgery* but only after the manuscript was retrieved from the garbage bin by the editors! This paper was also novel for using a disease-specific questionnaire to assess patients' arm function (Lokanathan et al. 2001).

When Tony was grumpy, he could be really grumpy. Nurses and residents would invariably avoid him on bad days. But grumpiness can be leveraged, and one of Tony's greatest contributions to the BC vascular surgeons was being our representative during fee negotiations. Tony was instrumental in elevating our billings from out of the doldrums. When only a minor increase was offered for a follow-up visit, Tony's response was: "I can't do anything with that." To

---

81   Thoracic outlet: space between collar bone and first rib through which the blood vessels and nerves to the arm pass.

82   Paget-Schroetter disease: clotting of vein underneath the collar bone.

83   Thrombolysis: process of actively dissolving blood clots using "clot busting" drugs.

which the government negotiators increased the amount to his (and our) satisfaction.

But, when he was happy and humming an Elvis tune, everything was fine. With his rich tenor voice, one of the nurses asked if his other job was in phone sex. And to hear him refer to a vascular horrendoma

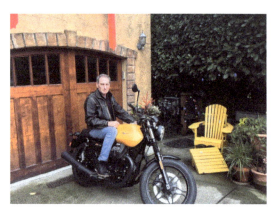

as a "blue plate special" and talk about patients and staff who could only "vibrate at a low frequency" brought a huge smile to all of us.

Dr. Diana Lynn Doyle, MD FRCSC

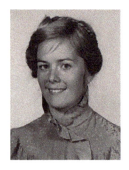

Dr. Lynn Doyle was the first vascular fellow of the UBC Vascular Surgery program, and when she graduated, she became the first female vascular surgeon in Canada. She was probably the least understood of all the fellows. Being female, blond, and petite, she could also swear like a truck driver, but had a heart of gold.

Lynn was a BC "lifer," receiving her MD, general surgery, and vascular surgery training all from UBC. After her vascular fellowship she spent time at Cedars Sinai Medical Centre in Los Angeles under the supervision of Dr. Warren Grundfest. Upon returning to Vancouver, she was appointed staff surgeon at UBCH with Wally Chung and Peter Fry.

Apart from clinical care, Lynn's interests in medicine lay in medical politics, where she quickly advanced from local hospital committees to the British Columbia Medical Association (now renamed *Doctors of BC*) where she continually rose, becoming their president in 2002. For the Division of Vascular Surgery, Lynn served as acting head from 2004 to 2007. With no further dragons to slay, Lynn chose early retirement in 2007.

Our careers overlapped as residents and later as staff. Lynn was one of my first senior residents in general surgery. I was impressed not only with her knowledge and dedication to surgery, but her ability to recognize strengths and weaknesses, both in herself and others. As a result, we got on very well. After I joined the UBCH staff in 1989, Lynn and I shared a clinical secretary. Lynn could be bullish to those she barely tolerated and did not suffer fools gladly. Nurses, students, and residents were terrified of her, but I found it just a cover for her fiery dedication to patient care. If the definition of a surgeon is a doctor who is "always right, never wrong, and never in doubt," then they must have been thinking of Lynn when they created the saying.

Dr. David Charles Taylor, MD, FRCSC

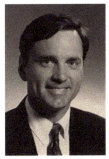 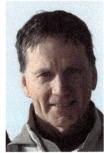 Dr. David Taylor was also a UBC product, having received his MD, general surgery, and vascular surgery training, all at UBC. Dave was mentored by all the vascular surgeons he met. From Henry Litherland, he learned leadership skills and calmness under pressure. From Henry

Hildebrand, he learned the need for compassion and excellence in surgical technique. From Peter Fry, he learned about complex surgical care.

After completing the vascular fellowship, he spent an additional year with Dr. Eugene Strandness in Seattle, learning about vascular ultrasound and all aspects of vascular surgery. Dr. Strandness taught him the need for meticulous research methods and became a lifelong mentor. One of the benefits of working in a first-class lab was meeting many outstanding young surgeons, many of whom would become future leaders in vascular surgery. One young surgeon, Greg Moneta, became fast friends with Dave. Of their many unique research projects, one stood out: to study the visceral ultrasound characteristics of different meals injected into the stomach, they placed nasogastric tubes in each other (Moneta et al. 1988). They had a willingness to do almost anything to get a research paper published!

Since then, Dave has spent his entire career at UBC. He has served as division head of Vascular Surgery, president of the Pacific Northwest Vascular Society and the Canadian Society of Vascular Surgery, and has had important education roles with the Vascular Surgery committee of the Royal College of Physicians and Surgeons of Canada, including chief examiner for Vascular Surgery. Despite these accolades, Dave's proudest achievement has been the many vascular surgeons he has helped train at UBC.

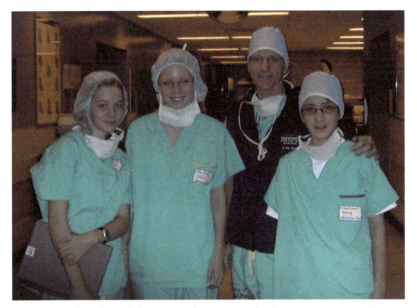

Dr. David Taylor with latest crop of junior Vascular Surgery trainees. c. 2004.

Dr. York N. Hsiang, MB ChB, MHSc, FRCSC

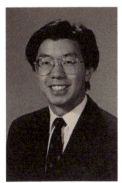 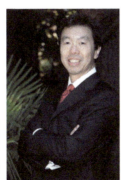

My only exposure to vascular surgery as a medical student was one lecture given by a radiologist. I recall that the room was stifling hot and dark, and the speaker droned on, showing umpteen black and white images of angiograms. No wonder I never considered it as a career. It was only during my time as a junior resident that I realized I needed to become a vascular surgeon. Up until that point, my surgical experience was limited to watching very average general surgeons (even I could tell!) fumble through their cases. But, meeting Henry Hildebrand in the OR was a revelation. Here was somebody worth emulating: decisive, incredibly fast but precise, and a gentleman. However, Henry was not the only one. As I met the other vascular surgeons, I discovered they were all cut from the same cloth.

I also learned that vascular surgery complications are highly unique. Peter Fry had to chew me out for going back to sleep after I was asked to see a herald bleed from a blown axillary artery anastomosis. By the time I saw the patient, the nurses had removed all the evidence, including the blood on the ceiling. Everything looked fine, and I went back to sleep. Surprisingly, that appropriate reaming out did not alter my view about vascular surgery. If anything, it made me more driven to become part of the club who did this type of dangerous surgery.

My first memories of becoming a staff surgeon at VGH in 1994 was like entering high school all over again. Despite completing my residency there, and having been a staff surgeon at UBCH for five years, the doctors and nurses remembered me as the young resident, and treated me as such for the better part of that first year. What I didn't realize was that I needed a breakthrough event to declare that I was no longer a resident.

That moment came later the same year when a local physician was brought in emergently with a gunshot wound in an attempted homicide. But this was no ordinary wound. Canada is a relatively peaceful society and the very limited gunshot wounds we see are almost all from handguns. This was an AK-47 wound, with a small entrance wound on the medial side of the lower thigh and an enormous exit wound on the lateral thigh. My patient was dying.

The OR was quickly prepared, and I went through the usual damage control of proximal and distal control of bleeding. There was at least a 5 to 7 cm section of shattered popliteal artery[84] and femoral vein. We prepped the opposite leg and harvested the contralateral great saphenous vein for the replacement conduit as recommended by all the textbooks. However, even fully distended, the great saphenous vein was minuscule, no more than 2 mm. So, at this juncture, our options were limited. We could force the small vein as the conduit, spend another hour harvesting the contralateral femoral vein, or use a prosthetic bypass, recognizing the high risk of graft infection and need for further surgery later.

By this time, we had been in the OR for several hours, having done an initial fasciotomy[85], spending time arresting the hemorrhage, digging out the saphenous vein and now this. We needed to revascularize his leg. So, I requested two PTFE grafts, one 6 mm and the other, 8 mm, to replace the blown-out artery and vein.

That day, somebody must have been looking out for me, because it worked. We had saved his leg, but most importantly, saved a physician from certain death. He required skin grafts and developed a pulmonary embolus[86] while in hospital, but was discharged home and continued to work after a period of rehabilitation. And the PTFE grafts? They never became infected and functioned for the next twenty years.

For me, the success of that case meant I had finally arrived. Doctors and nurses who knew me as a resident would stop and take the time to make small talk, like you'd do with a colleague. Since then, my career has been a stepwise progression to professor of

---

84   Popliteal artery: artery behind knee.
85   Fasciotomy: surgical procedure to cut through skin down to muscle.
86   Pulmonary embolus: blood clot that travels into lung.

surgery, UBC division head, lead of various committees, and president of the Western Vascular Surgery Society (the first Canadian to be so honoured). That case was the seminal event that opened the door to my career. When medical students ask me about how I chose vascular surgery, I tell them that life is fated, and "those who begin with doubts end in certainties" (adapted from Francis Bacon).

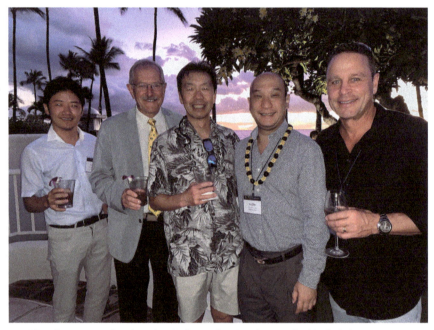

Vascular surgeons hard at play. Left to right: Keisuke Miyake (Osaka), Steve Murray (Spokane), YNH, Yiu-che Chan (Hong Kong), Ben Starnes (Seattle). c. 2019.

Dr. Jerry C. Chen, MD, MSc, FRCSC

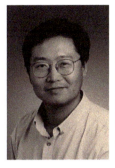 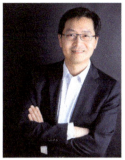 Dr. Jerry Chen received his basic medical and general surgery training from the University of Manitoba before coming to Vancouver as the first Rogers fellow in 1995. During his tenure, I discovered that he had "green thumbs"—whatever he planted, grew! This was the most academically productive period of our program, having a dedicated research fellow and regular weekly research meetings. His productivity resulted in many publications, and led to his MSc degree during this period.

After the completion of his fellowship, Jerry undertook additional training with visiting fellowship positions at Harbor-UCLA (Dr. Rodney White) and the University of Hong Kong (Dr. Stephen Cheng). He was recruited back to VGH in 1998 to replace Henry Hildebrand.

Since then, Jerry's career has been on an upward spiral, serving as program director twice, as UBC and VGH division head of Vascular Surgery, and as a Royal College examiner in vascular surgery. I have long appreciated his "can do" attitude and fearlessness. From burying himself in completely new research projects to recognizing the need to acquire new skills (like me, Jerry undertook a mini endovascular fellowship in 2006), and taking on controversial administrative positions that none of us wanted (his second tenure as program director was a raucous affair over the placement of residents at the teaching hospitals), Jerry's laid back style is a testament to those of us who want proof that it's possible to appear calm when treading water—nothing's happening above the water line but below, your arms and legs are moving like crazy!

Dr. Joel J. Gagnon, MD, FRCSC

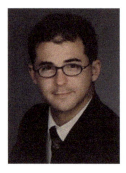

In the early 2000s, we had a flurry of fellows from Quebec. Dr. Joel Gagnon was the first, and we were asked by his Laval University chief, Dr. Yvan Douville, to "keep our mitts off him" as he was meant to return to Laval to do great things. We had no idea what extraordinary talents lay in Quebec.

Joel was the youngest of our fellows who trained at UBC, owing to a two-year college diploma program that served as a pre-med requirement in Quebec (unlike a four-year undergraduate degree program required elsewhere in Canada). He received his MD and general surgery training at Laval University before driving across the country to start his vascular fellowship in BC.

Coming out west was also an opportunity for Joel to improve his English. I felt he was particularly brave to ignore all the snickering about his Franco-English. At times, however, the nuances of language would get him into trouble. For example, in French, there is no word that ends in *th*. The closest way of pronouncing this would have it end in *t*. This was borne out when on rounds one morning, a female carotid patient was shocked when Joel asked her to smile and show her teet(h)!

Nonetheless, the language of surgery came naturally to Joel. After completing the UBC vascular fellowship, he pursued additional endovascular fellowships in Groningen, in the Netherlands, Nuremburg, and Melbourne.

Coming from a farming background, Joel also had great skills in the kitchen and outdoors. Fishing was one of his innate abilities; he always managed to catch all the fish.

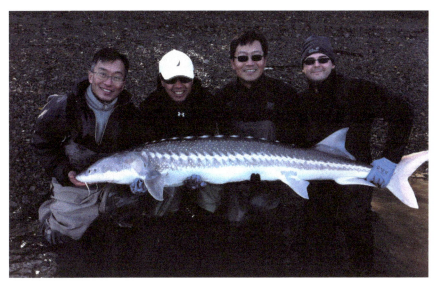

Sturgeon fishing with the boys. Left to right: Stanley Tung, YNH, Jerry Chen, Joel Gagnon.
c. 2011.

With the waterways conquered, he set his sights on the skies and pursued flying as a hobby. We honoured our commitment to not poach Joel from Laval, but life had different ideas. Joel met an OR nurse, got married, and decided to live in BC. Laval's loss was our gain, and Joel joined the VGH staff in 2007 to replace Lynn Doyle. He was a fearless surgeon, and soon 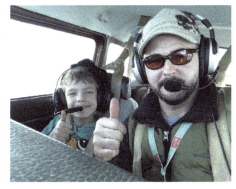 developed a well-deserved reputation as one of the primary endo-vascular surgeons for the province. Despite this, he was frustrated with the chronic shortage of resources at VGH, and in 2019 he left for the Royal Columbia Hospital in New Westminster, BC.

Dr. Keith A. Baxter, MSc, MD, FRCSC

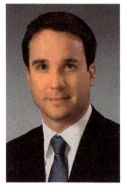

Dr. Keith Baxter grew up in Vancouver and attended the same school as Dave Taylor, but a decade later. In university, he was interested in science and completed an MSc in anatomy before entering UBC Medical School. It was on a vascular surgery rotation that he was bitten by the vascular surgery bug and entered the UBC general surgery program followed by the vascular fellowship.

It was during his general surgery research time that I, as his co-supervisor, became aware of Keith's technical abilities as a microvascular surgeon. His project was to study the myogenic[87] effects of acid on rat coronary vessels, an extraordinarily challenging feat even using a dissecting microscope (Baxter et al. 2006).

During his fellowship he met his future wife, Tanya, a young ophthalmologist whose parents hailed from Australia. Many things Australian followed. After completion of his vascular fellowship, he received additional endovascular training in Melbourne and Sydney. Tanya and Keith also named their son Jackson, partially as an acknowledgement of the original name for Sydney, Australia.

Since returning to UBC to replace Peter Fry, Keith's even personality has led to progressive administrative positions including program director, division head, and most recently surgeon-in-chief at VGH.

---

87 Myogenic: muscle.

Dr. Jason Faulds, MD, MHSc, FRCSC

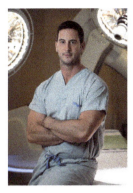

Dr. Jason Faulds came to Vancouver from Ontario, being born and raised in Northwestern Ontario. Jason attended medical school at Queen's University in Kingston, Ontario, and came west to pursue a general surgery residency at UBC. During this residency Jason completed a master's degree in health sciences, with a focus on clinical epidemiology. Following this, Jason did his vascular surgery fellowship at UBC and subsequently a fellowship in open thoracic aortic surgery at the University of Texas, under the guidance of Dr. Hazim Safi, a world-renowned cardiothoracic surgeon. Jason returned to Vancouver in 2015 as a consultant vascular surgeon with a special interest in thoracic aortic disease.

Jason is a proud parent of four young children and a wonderful golden retriever named Hercules. When not operating or parenting you might catch him fly fishing, deer hunting, or kiteboarding. He is also a proud third line grinder on his beer league hockey team.

Dr. Jonathan Misskey, MD, MHPE, FRCSC

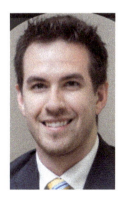

Our most recently appointed surgeon, Dr. Jon Misskey, hails from Saskatchewan. He completed two years of ecology from 2006–8 at the University of Regina before entering the University of Saskatchewan where he obtained his MD in 2016. Jon was our first direct entry resident in the 2012 vascular surgery match. We discovered he had a real passion for medical education; he enrolled in an education enrichment program, ultimately obtaining a masters in health professions education from the University of Maastricht in 2016. Jon completed his residency in vascular surgery in 2019 and was recruited to replace Joel Gagnon, who departed for Royal Columbian Hospital the same year. In 2020, he was appointed as program director.

During his time as a resident, Jon demonstrated considerable academic prowess and was the first author of two manuscripts describing the management of access-related hand ischemia (Misskey et al. 2015), and optimizing arteriovenous fistula patency[88] (Misskey et al. 2020). The former paper was recognized as an important contribution to vascular access and featured in the 2018 Clinical Practice Guidelines for the European Society for Vascular Access (EJVS 2018). The latter paper was selected by the editors of the *Journal of Vascular Surgery* for a special commentary by Dr. Thomas Huber, who agreed with the paper's proposed treatment algorithm to optimize fistula patency (Huber 2020).

Surviving residency is difficult for all, but getting married and having a child during residency can be even more challenging. Not to be outdone, Jon and his wife, Anna, managed to produce a set of twin girls during his residency. One could say their lives are very full now!

---

88   Arteriovenous fistula: surgical procedure to connect an artery to a vein, usually used in hemodialysis.

PART SIX

GRADUATES OF THE VASCULAR SURGERY PROGRAM

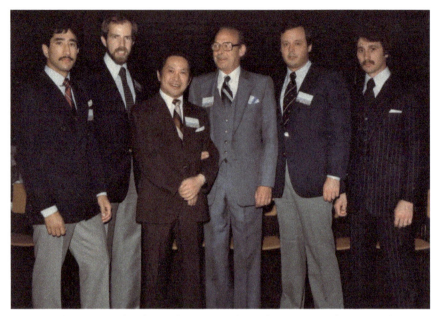

UBC residents and staff. Left to Right: Gene Zierler, Mike Janusz (Cardiac Surgery), Wally Chung, Frank Patterson (Surgery Dept. Head), Tony Dow (General Surgery), Tony Salvian. c. 1981.

The lifeline of any graduate program is its fellows and residents. The UBC program is very proud of its graduates, all of whom have gone on to have excellent surgical careers. Some went further and blossomed into medical and academic leaders. The following are the graduates who successfully completed the program from 1981 to 2020. Many attempts were made to contact the graduates, but from the majority there was no response; thus the unequal length of the following entries. I like to think the lives and practices of all of our graduates are rewarding and productive.

R. Eugene Zierler, MD (1980–1981)

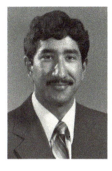 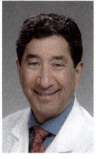

"I graduated from the Johns Hopkins University School of Medicine in May 1976, and started my general surgery residency at VGH in July. As a medical student, I had very little exposure to the specialty we now refer to as *vascular surgery*, but I had developed a special interest in cardiovascular physiology, and my intent was to finish general surgery training and pursue additional training in cardiac surgery. My wife at that time was from British Columbia, and after visiting Vancouver several times as a medical student, I made the somewhat unusual decision (for an American) to apply for a residency position at UBC.

My first rotation at VGH was on a general surgery service that included several busy vascular surgeons: Dr. Henry Hildebrand, who had been practising for many years, and Dr. Peter Fry, who was a relative newcomer to the faculty. The other vascular surgeons at VGH in those days were Dr. Wally Chung and Dr. Henry Litherland. The general surgeons on that service, as best I can recall, were Dr. A. D. McKenzie, Dr. Ted Robbins, and Dr. Leonard Fratkin. The senior residents on that service were interested in the "big" general surgery cases—Whipple's, gastrectomies, hepatic resections, and the like, so as the most recent addition, I ended up as the only resident scrubbed on a lot of the vascular cases. Dr. Hildebrand was an especially gifted technical surgeon and working with him in the operating room was an eye-opening experience. I found the vascular procedures extremely interesting, both from the technical and physiological points of view. As I gained more experience, I discovered that I had some innate technical ability for vascular surgery, and Dr. Hildebrand generously let me operate quite a bit, even as a first-year resident. Over a number of months and subsequent rotations, I realized that I was developing a serious interest in vascular surgery and started to consider the possibility that this would be worth pursuing as an alternative to cardiac surgery.

One night early in my first year, while I was on duty, I went to the VGH library to do some reading about vascular surgery. In 1976, there were not many books dedicated to that specialty, but there was one on the shelf entitled *Hemodynamics for Surgeons* by D. Eugene Strandness and David S. Sumner. I found this book immensely interesting, and it addressed many of the questions I was starting to ask about vascular disease and vascular surgery procedures. It described a physiological approach to the diagnosis and treatment of vascular abnormalities, combining basic science, engineering, medicine, and surgery. These were the basic features of cardiac physiology and surgery that had appealed to me as a medical student. This book also introduced me to the concept of non-invasive vascular testing, something that would soon play an important role in my career.

Around the time that I began my training at VGH, Dr. Fry and the vascular surgeons had just started a vascular diagnostic laboratory. The instrumentation available at that time included continuous-wave Doppler and some type of plethysmography that could be used to measure segmental limb pressures, and obtain flow waveforms and volume pulses. The most sophisticated device in the new vascular laboratory was called an *ultrasonic arteriograph*, which was a rather complicated pulsed Doppler imaging system built by the D. E. Hokanson company. This allowed the examiner to generate a "flow image" of the carotid bifurcation and obtain Doppler waveforms from the imaged vessels. Although this device worked as intended, it was difficult to use, and it would be superseded by duplex scanning a few years later. However, we learned a lot from using the ultrasonic arteriograph, and I later recognized that it was an important stepping stone in the development of duplex ultrasound.

By the time my second year of training started, I had essentially forgotten about cardiac surgery and was focusing on vascular surgery as I continued my general surgery training. Based on my rapidly expanding interest in vascular surgery and the vascular laboratory, Dr. Fry suggested that I spend some time in Seattle at the University of Washington in the laboratory of Dr. D. Eugene Strandness, who was a vascular surgeon and leader in the relatively new field of non-invasive vascular testing. Coincidentally, Dr. Strandness was also the lead author of the hemodynamics book that had made such an impression on me the previous year (by this time, I had obtained my own copy and read all 657 pages). The plan was for me to visit the Strandness laboratory and then come back to VGH and help develop the vascular laboratory there.

I arrived at the Strandness laboratory at the University of Washington Medical Center in the fall of 1978 and stayed until the spring of 1979. At our first meeting, after some introductions, Dr. Strandness escorted me down the hall from his office to a large room filled with electronic equipment and bins of electronic parts. In the middle of the room were several racks of electronic components and a table with a thin mattress and a small pillow. He described this as the new duplex ultrasound scanner that was being built by the bioengineers and told me that I would be using this instrument to evaluate patients with carotid artery disease. The rest, as the saying goes, is history.

My overall experience in the Strandness laboratory in 1978–1979 was, to say the least, life changing. I not only learned a great deal about ultrasound and vascular disease, but also started to think seriously about how to approach clinical problems, work as part of a research team, write scientific papers, and present research findings. Dr. Strandness and I seemed to get along well, and when I returned to Vancouver, he left an open invitation for me to come back to Seattle.

From July 1979 through June 1981, I finished my general surgery residency at UBC. As I recall, the three most common operations on my list as a chief resident were cholecystectomy, colon resection, and femoral-popliteal bypass. I also kept in touch with Dr. Strandness throughout this period, and continued to work on projects and write papers based on my initial experience in his laboratory. When I finished my general surgery residency in 1981, I submitted a successful application for an associate investigator award based at the Seattle VA Medical Center and returned to Seattle to continue my work in the Strandness laboratory and pursue further training in vascular surgery at the University of Washington. In those days, there were no accredited fellowships in vascular surgery, and recognition of vascular surgery as a distinct surgical specialty was still years away, so a "fellowship" was whatever you could arrange at an institution where there was expertise and a willingness to teach. With support from my associate investigator award, I was able to spend the next two years as both a clinical and research fellow under the mentorship of Dr. Brian Thiele, who was chief of the Vascular Surgery section at the Seattle VA Medical Center, and Dr. Strandness at the University of Washington.

When I finished my vascular surgery training in 1983, there were no faculty positions open at the University of Washington, so I accepted a position at the Wadsworth (West Los Angeles) VA Medical Center at UCLA where I had the opportunity to establish my own vascular laboratory and was the only formally trained vascular surgeon. But my time in Los Angeles turned out to be relatively brief. Shortly after I left Seattle, Dr. Thiele decided to move to the Penn State Hershey Medical Center, and I was asked by Dr. Strandness to fill his position at the Seattle VA Medical Center, which I was glad to do. So, in 1984, I returned to Seattle for the third time, and I have been on the University of Washington faculty continuously since that time.

Looking back on these events, I am extremely grateful for the rich vascular surgery and vascular laboratory experience I had during my years of training at UBC. The trust and encouragement I received from the original vascular surgeons at VGH were major factors in putting me on the professional path I am still on today. I have managed to be in the right place at the right time to participate in many important developments, and I have tried to take full advantage of the opportunities that have been presented to me. Dr. Strandness became a lifelong friend and colleague, and it has been a privilege to continue the work he started here at the University of Washington."

Dr. James Dooner, MD FRCSC, FACS (1982)

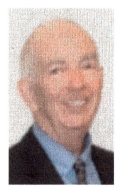

Dr. Jim Dooner obtained his MD from the University of Western Ontario in 1976, followed by residency in general and vascular surgery at UBC. He provided vascular surgical care to the Victoria, BC community from 1982 to 2016. Jim's varied leadership positions included chief of surgery for Vancouver Island Health Authority, head of the Division of Vascular Surgery at the Royal Jubilee Hospital, president of the CSVS, and member of the board of directors of the SVS.

In 2001, he received an MBA from the University of Victoria. As a result of the new knowledge and skills related to business education, Jim trained and obtained certification in Discrete Event Simulation, as well as Lean Design for Healthcare and Lean Design for the OR from the University of Tennessee. Jim is happily retired and spends his days rowing, reading, and playing guitar.

Dr. Annette Holmvang (1986–1987)

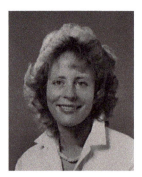

Dr. Annette Holmvang is a Vancouver native and UBC product, having received her MD and fellowships in general and vascular surgery from UBC. She was the second female fellow and after completing her fellowship, practised in Richmond, BC with Gord Houston. She is retired and enjoys spending time with her family.

Dr. Jock Reid (1986–1987)

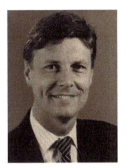

Before he became a doctor, Dr. Jock Reid was a teacher. Perhaps the students finally got to him, or the proverbial light went on. Jock received his MD from the University of Calgary and came west to complete his general and vascular surgery training at UBC. During his time as a resident, trauma surgery was his passion and Jock developed into one of the first surgical residents to become an ATLS instructor. Trauma surgery carried him to Parkland Hospital, Dallas for post fellowship training.

After his time in Dallas, Jock returned to UBC and has practised since then at SPH. He has served as the SPH Division head of Vascular Surgery, and is the current SPH Department of Surgery head. In his spare time, Jock enjoys running and indulging his daughters' passion for horses.

Dr. Luis Rosada-Lopez (1987–1988)

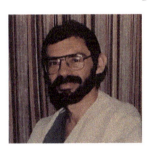

Originally from Mexico, Dr. Lopez was a cardiac surgery resident when he decided to do additional training in vascular surgery. He was highly technically competent, but also had a fiery streak. Luis is believed to currently be in the United States.

Dr. Aristotle Azad (1988–1989)

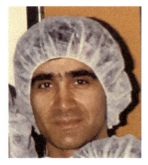

Dr. Aristotle Azad was an MD and PhD (Anatomy) student at UBC before entering general surgery residency. Initially, he was drawn to pediatric general surgery because of his good friend, Chris Moir (Chris would go on to become a pediatric general surgeon at the Mayo Clinic). However, Aris was strongly influenced by the swashbuckling Peter Fry, and changed his career goal to vascular surgery. After completing his vascular fellowship, he moved to Kamloops, BC, where he has practised ever since. When not in the OR, Aris can be found in the many surrounding mountains.

Dr. Michael Riggs (1988–1989)

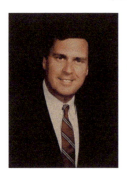

Dr. Michael Riggs was our first vascular fellow from the United States. Mike was from Oklahoma, and true to the nature of southern Americans, was a gentleman and a cool customer, both in and out of the OR. After finishing his fellowship, Mike returned to Oklahoma where he practised his entire career. He enjoyed introducing others to his passion for cars, especially "sleepers" that could burn rubber in every gear. Soon after finishing, Mike sent me a photo of his fifteen-bedroom mansion in Oklahoma. The cost of it was about the price of a small condo in Vancouver.

Dr. Suvro Sett (1989)

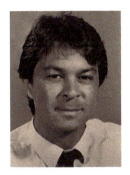

Dr. Suvro Sett was a UBC cardiac surgery resident who completed the vascular fellowship. Suvro introduced the use of micro instruments to the staff at UBCH, although the quality of our instruments at the time was substandard.

After completing his fellowship, Suvro was appointed as a pediatric cardiac surgeon at BC Children's Hospital before relocating to the United States to continue his career there.

Dr. David Ratliff (1989–1990)

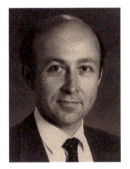

Dr. (or Mr.) David Ratliff came to Vancouver from the UK in 1989, already an accomplished general surgeon with an interest in endocrine, transplant, and vascular surgery. Facetiously, we thought he came for his "BTC" degree, i.e., "Been to Canada." He was particularly interested in new technology, and was in the right place at the right time as his fellowship experience coincided with much of the early endovascular development at UBCH.

After completing his fellowship, he returned to the UK, working at Leicester Royal Infirmary from 1991–94 before moving to Northampton General Hospital, where he has led the progressive development and delivery of the general, endocrine, and vascular surgical services.

Dr. Mussaad Al-Salman, (1989–1991)

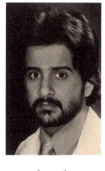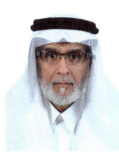

Dr. Mussaad Al-Salman was born in Riyadh, Saudi Arabia. After graduating from the King Saud University School of Medicine, in Saudi Arabia, Mussaad came to Canada to receive higher education in general and vascular surgery.

He returned to Riyadh after completion of his vascular fellowship, and was appointed medical director of the Accident and Emergency Department of the King Khalid University Hospital. His career has been on a rapid trajectory since then, with appointments as professor of surgery and Chair of the Department of Surgery at King Saud University, followed by Vice Dean for Hospital Affairs, Dean of the College of Medicine (all at King Saud University), and Vice Rector for Health Affairs at the Princess Nora Bint Rahman University.

Mussaad's outstanding career has demonstrated considerable pioneering vision—he was also the founder and head of the Division of Vascular Surgery and the Vascular Laboratory at the King Khalid University Hospital, as well as the founder and chair of the King Saud University Vascular Surgery fellowship.

Dr. Hamid Nasser (1990–1991)

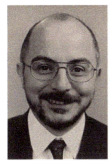 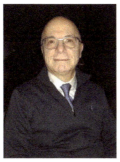

Dr. Hamid Nasser was originally from Lebanon. The following are his recollections:

"I started my training in the UBC vascular surgery fellowship program in July 1990, after completing a general surgery residency at the Université de Montréal. Dr. Peter Fry was the program director and my mentor at UBC.

Following the completion of my fellowship, my first job was in New Glasgow, Nova Scotia (NS) at the Aberdeen Hospital, where I did general and vascular surgery until 1994. I then moved to the Valley Regional Hospital in Kentville, NS, for a year, after which I moved to Dr. Everett Chalmers Hospital in Fredericton, New Brunswick. I wanted to move to Ontario where my wife had family; however, Ontario was not licensing physicians who were not trained in Ontario.

In 1996, Ontario changed the rules of licensing which allowed me to move to the Humber River Regional Hospital in 1996. The workload became difficult to manage, mainly because I was the only vascular surgeon providing coverage for two sites, and I was still doing both general and vascular surgery.

I moved to the Guelph General Hospital in Guelph, Ontario, in 2002, and dedicated my practice to vascular surgery. Eventually, I completed a mini-fellowship in endovascular surgery with Dr. Marc Bosiers at AZ Saint-Blasius Hospital in Dendermonde, Belgium in 2006. Following that mini-fellowship, I established the endovascular program at the Guelph General Hospital with a hybrid room. It has since become the regional vascular surgery program.

My vivid memory about UBC is that early in my training, I was doing my evening rounds around seven o'clock in the evening, when Dr. Peter Fry happened to walk by, and he asked me what I was still doing in the hospital. When I told him that I was doing my evening rounds, he told me without hesitation, "Go home to your wife; it is getting late." This may sound benign to any reader; however, I had just finished a residency in general surgery in Montreal where the program treated you more like a slave than a resident (no doubt things have changed since). So, to me, being treated like a human being was a drastic change, and this approach applied to all the staff at UBC during the time I spent with them.

I'm proud to have been trained under all of them."

Dr. Roman Huhlewych (1991–1992)

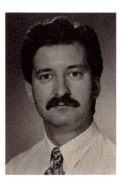

Dr. Roman Huhlewych came from Ontario, and returned there after completing his vascular fellowship. Roman currently practises in Scarborough, ON.

Dr. Ghaith Khougheer (1991–1992)

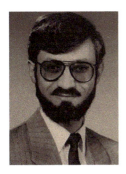

Dr. Ghaith Khougheer graduated from the King Abdulla Medical School in Saudi Arabia before coming to Vancouver for general and vascular surgery training. After completing the vascular fellowship, Ghaith returned to Saudi Arabia and initially practised at Aramco Hospital in Dhahran, before moving, in 2016, to the Johns Hopkins Aramco Health Care Speciality Clinics, where he continues to work.

Dr. Jim Hunter (1992–1993)

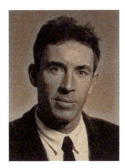

Dr. Jim Hunter was first a lawyer before becoming a doctor. He received his basic medical, general, and vascular surgery training, all at UBC. Jim practised general and vascular surgery at the Lions Gate Hospital in North Vancouver until he retired in 2018.

Dr. Gordon Houston (1993–1994)

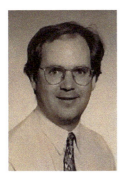

Dr. Gordon Houston was another "UBC lifer" who received his medical and specialist training at UBC. Gord practices general and vascular surgery in Richmond, BC.

Dr. Sameh Barayan (1994–1995)

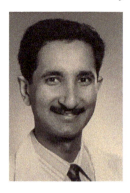

Unlike many other Saudi trainees, Dr. Sameh Barayan was extremely confident, and not shy when expressing his opinions. We called him "The Prince" because of his regal mannerisms. After finishing the fellowship, Sameh returned to Aramco in Saudi Arabia, and worked there before entering private practice.

Dr. Gregory Lewis (1995–1996)

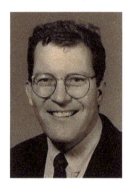

Dr. Greg Lewis was from Cape Town, South Africa, and he received his medical and general surgery training there. He immigrated with his family to BC, and practised as a family physician in northern BC until he entered the vascular fellowship. Greg practises general and vascular surgery in Abbotsford, BC.

Dr. Robert Turnbull (1996–1998)

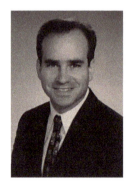

Dr. Robert Turnbull was the first of our Edmonton-trained general surgeons who came to Vancouver for their vascular fellowship. I thought he was a dog lover since a lot of his comments referred to "puppies," as in: "let's take care of those puppies." His other favourite comment was "Let's get out of Dodge," as a hint that we should close up and conclude the operation, as his caffeine levels were falling. He was the only fellow I met who would have a can of Coke for breakfast.

Acronyms were slowly being added to our lexicons, and Rob introduced us to the best-known Edmonton acronym, FUFA, otherwise affectionately known as a *fucked up femoral artery*. FUFAs must have been common in Edmonton, since Rob had many stories of how he encountered FUFAs of different sizes under varying conditions.

Some residents have terrible call karma—whenever you took call with them, you knew it was going to be an all-nighter. With Rob, I thought he had good call karma until I spent a weekend doing three ruptured AAAs with him. No other resident or fellow has ever come close to that. After completion of the vascular fellowship, Robert returned to Edmonton, where he remains in vascular surgery practice today.

Dr. Albert Ting (1998)

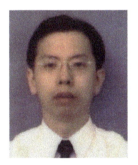

Dr. Albert Ting was the first Hong Kong trainee recommended by his chief, Dr. Stephen Cheng, to receive vascular surgery training at UBC (see "The Hong Kong Connection"). Here are his thoughts on his training:

"I was privileged to be able to work as a vascular fellow in the Division of Vascular Surgery at UBC between July and December 1998 under the supervision of Professors York Hsiang and David Taylor. At that time, I had just finished general surgery training at the Department of Surgery of the University of Hong Kong at Queen Mary Hospital, and started specializing in vascular surgery. It was a great experience with much hands-on training opportunities in vascular surgery procedures, including endovascular stent graft repair of aneurysms. I also took the opportunity to join the laboratory of Professor Hsiang to learn some basic research techniques and methodology.

During the [fellowship], I was able to attend the Western Vascular Society's annual meeting in Whistler, BC. It was an eye-opening experience to attend a great vascular conference with many renowned experts in the field.

On the whole, the fellowship was a great experience and it was a great privilege to train with the vascular group at UBC. I will treasure their friendship forever.

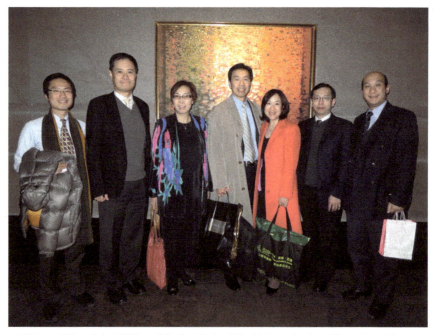

Visiting HK and the HKU staff. Left to Right, Alfred Wong, Stephen Cheng, Roz Chung, YNH, Bev Hsiang, Albert Ting, Yiu-che Chan. c. 2013.

Dr. Gerrit Winkelaar (1997–1999)

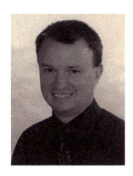

Dr. Gerrit Winkelaar, who followed his friend and colleague, Rob Turnbull, introduced us to more Edmonton sayings, such as "So, you want to be a vascular surgeon?" This gem was used specifically when you were elbow deep in trouble. His other famous term was "audible bleeding."

Like Rob Turnbull, Gerrit graduated from the University of Alberta and received general surgery training there. Gerrit was the first polymath I have encountered in medicine. There was no topic too mundane, no date too obscure, and no sporting event too trivial—he knew it all by heart.

After completing his fellowship, Gerrit practised for a short time at Royal Columbian Hospital before returning to Edmonton where he has served as the Division head of Vascular Surgery, president of the CSVS, and president of the Alberta Medical Association.

He enjoys travelling and mountain climbing (ask him about the Himalayas) with his wife, Robin, while trying to spend all his money before his kids can get their share.

Dr. Arthur Chan (1999-2000)

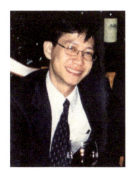

Dr. Arthur Chan was the second Hong Kong fellow, after Albert Ting. Arthur graduated from the University of Hong Kong and received his general surgery training at Princess Margaret Hospital, Hong Kong.

As the vascular fellow, his first rotation was at SPH, and the staff decided to entertain Arthur with a few drinks in order to loosen him up. Surprising to them, Arthur had no trouble handling the amount of alcohol provided and proceeded to drink the SPH staff under the table. A legend was instantly born. He recalls his time in BC:

"I was thrilled to hear that Professor Hsiang was going to write about the vascular fellowship program, and I feel privileged to have this chance to share my experience, dating back to October 1999. And as I start recalling, it seems just like yesterday.

I was, I believe, the second HK participant to join the program. With the kind recommendation by Professor Steven Cheng, I got the chance to follow in the steps of Dr. Albert Ting, about half a year after his term. There was a big difference between Albert and me. Albert was already an experienced vascular surgeon when he joined the program, and I was just a green surgeon in the field. I was working in a peripheral hospital in Kowloon (Princess Margaret Hospital, PMH) and I had the mission to reinforce the vascular service after my short half-year training. I have to give my whole-hearted thanks to all the surgeons and staff involved in the program (VGH, SPH, UBCH) who gave me huge support.

During the program, I had ample cutting experiences, both as assistant and as chief surgeon. All the staff shared with me their tricks, with no reservation. All aspects of vascular surgery were covered from thoracoabdominal aneurysm repair, ruptured AAA repair, aorto-enteric bypass, carotid endarterectomy, lower limb revascularization, dialysis vascular access, and vein surgery. I also had a chance to attend cases less commonly seen in HK, such as chronic compartment syndrome, cervical rib resection, etc.

I was also given the chance to attend vein clinics (and perform sclerotherapy), angiogram meetings, journal clubs, and a three-day vascular workshop held in Santa Monica for vascular fellows, through which I gained much experience to share with my co-workers at PMH.

Last but not the least, I learned to give loving care to patients and their relatives, and to deal with their emotions (for instance, helping an old lady to accept an AKA, and a renal failure patient to accept a redo AVF).

After my training, with great support from my consultant mentor, Dr. L. S. Ho, I helped reorganize the vascular service in my hospital and establish the vascular laboratory to improve vascular diagnosis. We also started carotid screening and carotid endarterectomy. I shared all the tricks I learned from my UBC teachers with my team members, and we subsequently also expanded the service to include endovascular surgery.

I entered private practice as a general surgeon in 2005, and am now doing mainly general surgery. However, my experience from vascular training has given me a lot of confidence. After all, the basis of surgery is anatomy, especially vascular anatomy. The book *Comprehensive Vascular Exposures* by Ronald J. Stoney is still my invaluable reference book. Vascular access (AVF creation, HD catheter, and portocath insertion) are still a significant part of my daily practice.

The short period in Vancouver as a visiting vascular fellow is certainly one of the best moments in my career. I still remember the happiness of participating in three ruptured aneurysm operations in a row, during a long weekend call; and of course, the delicious sushi dinner with my colleague (Dr. Ramesh Lokanathan). I have to thank Professor Hsiang and Dr. Jock Reid for inviting us for dinner during Thanksgiving and Christmas, and Dr. David Taylor for allowing us to visit his house in Whistler, where I learned to ski. I also will never forget the operating tricks of Dr. Lynn Doyle, Peter Fry, Tony Sylvian, Jerry Chen, and Shaun McDonald. Shaun was a new staff surgeon in SPH at the time and we had great times together, both at and after work. On my last day, Ramesh and Louis saw me off at the airport, and gave me a CD by Stompin' Tom Conners as a gift. It is still with me ("Tillsonburg" is my favourite song).

Finally, let me wish the program continued growth in the future, such that more surgeons can benefit from it."

Dr. Ramesh Lokanathan (1998–2000)

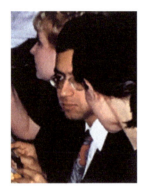 Dr. Ramesh Lokanathan graduated from McGill University and completed his general surgery training there before coming to UBC for the vascular fellowship. He was a quiet, kind soul, so you can imagine my surprise when he told me that, in his younger days, he had ultra-long hair, and was part of a punk rock band. At the time, I was in the habit of asking each graduating fellow to leave me a CD of their favourite music so I could listen to it while doing surgery and remember the times we had together. I got wonderful pieces. Gerrit Winkelaar introduced me to "music to drive by" featuring John Cougar Mellencamp. Peter Skaarsgard (a general surgery resident who went into cardiac surgery) got me hooked on jazz. David Kopriva sent me classical pieces. But when Ramesh left me a CD of his favourite punk rock music, I stopped the tradition. I had met my match. After completing vascular surgery training, Ramesh set up practice in Prince George, BC, where he remains today.

Dr. Renny Yien (2000)

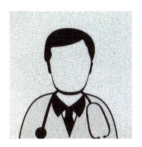

Dr. Renny Yien was the third Hong Kong fellow. He graduated from the University of Hong Kong and received his general surgery training at Ruttonjee Hospital, Hong Kong. Renny was adept at many things, and we all marvelled at his precision in using a nerve hook to tighten sutures. He also loved high-adrenalin sports and still continues with his diving adventures. After Renny returned to Hong Kong, he took up private practice in vascular surgery.

Dr. Louis Palerme (1999–2001)

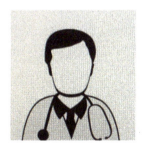

Dr. Louis Palerme was a bookend to Ramesh Lokanathan, both graduating from McGill and doing their general surgery training there. Like Ramesh, Louis was quiet and introspective. But when he introduced us to his favourite Prince lyrics, "Go crazy," which he applied to most things, I knew there must be a wild man inside of him. After finishing the vascular fellowship, Louis joined Ramesh and continues to practice in Prince George, BC.

Dr. David Kopriva (2000–2002)

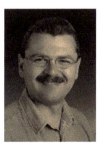

Dr. David Kopriva is currently a vascular surgeon in Regina, Saskatchewan, where he is also clinical assistant professor in the Department of Surgery, and adjunct professor in the College of Graduate Studies and Research at the University of Saskatchewan.

Upon completion of his medical degree at McGill University in Montreal, David continued with an internship at Royal Columbian Hospital in New Westminster in 1992. After two years of practising family medicine in New Westminster, he completed his residency in general surgery at the University of Saskatchewan. UBC Vascular Surgery welcomed him as a fellow in 2000. His accomplishments since then include certification as a "Lean Leader," and graduate of the advanced training program in health care delivery improvement offered at the Intermountain Healthcare Leadership Institute in Salt Lake City, Utah. This has led to the role of physician co-lead on the Saskatchewan Appropriateness of Care Initiative. Along the way, David has earned his pilot's licence, and he writes music, does research, works on clinical quality improvement projects, and most importantly, he has raised seven wonderful children with his wife, Patricia.

Dr. Shung Lee (2001–2003)

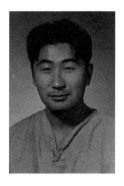

Dr. Shung Lee graduated from the University of Alberta before travelling west to BC for training in general and vascular surgery. Following graduation, Shung started practice in Victoria, BC, with Jim Dooner and colleagues. Since then, he has risen to division head of Vascular Surgery at Royal Jubilee Hospital. In his downtime, Shung enjoys fast activities such as hockey and driving.

Dr. Matt Smith (2002–2004)

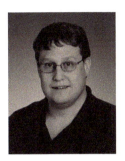

Dr. Matt Smith was another UBC lifer. After his fellowship, Matt initially practised in Calgary, AB, before returning to BC to practice in Abbotsford.

Dr. Dhafer Kamal (2003–2005)

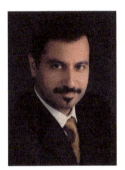

Dr. Dhafer Kamal came from Bahrain and received his medical training there. He went to McGill University for general surgery training before coming to UBC for the vascular fellowship. Since returning to Bahrain, Dhafer is now a senior consultant in vascular and endovascular surgery at BDF Hospital, Bahrain. He is also associate professor of surgery at the Royal College of Surgeons of Ireland and has served as the president of the Bahrain Vascular Association.

Dr. Edward Hui (2004)

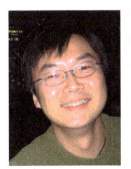

Dr. Edward Hui was our fourth and final fellow from Hong Kong. Edward received his medical degree from the University of Hong Kong, and general surgery training at Caritas Medical Centre, Hong Kong. He recalls his fellowship experiences:

"I came over in July 2004 and started with Drs. Reid, Macdonald, and Sidhu at SPH for three months. Since I was the only vascular trainee there, I saw almost every emergency admission. Such a vast amount of clinical exposure was a real eye opener.

Then I switched to VGH in October to learn from Dr. Chen, Dr. Salvian, Dr. Fry, Dr. Doyle, Dr. Taylor, and Dr. Hsiang. I trained alongside the other fellows, Dr. Dhafer Kamal from the Middle East, and Dr. Joel Gagnon, sharing vascular call. At VGH, I learned various operative techniques from different mentors.

At that time, open surgery was still the mainstay and endovascular surgery was still budding. It was a great time for me to have plenty of hands-on experience in open vascular surgery, laying a strong foundation for my practice when I returned to Hong Kong.

The six months of training was a very pleasant and fruitful experience, both clinically and socially. Now I am working in Ruttonjee Hospital in Hong Kong, as the chief of service in the Department of Surgery, providing service for both vascular and general surgery. I am really looking forward to visiting Vancouver again and had plans to come over this Christmas, but with COVID it seems that the plan has to be deferred."

Dr. Mohammed Al Assiri (2004–2006)

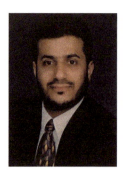

Dr. Mohammed Al Assiri (not be confused with the Saudi football player) was a quiet person and our fellow from 2004–06. After completing the vascular fellowship, he returned to Saudi Arabia where he currently works with another one of our fellows, Dr. Musaad Alghamdi, at the King Khalid University.

Dr. Hao Wu (2006–2008)

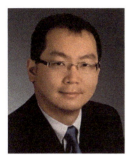

Dr. Hao Wu graduated from the University of Toronto and came to UBC for his fellowship. After its completion, he initially practised at Tufts Medical Center in Boston before relocating to Odessa, TX, where he remains in practice.

Dr. Marlene Grenon (2007–2009)

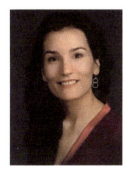

Dr. Marlene Grenon joined the vascular fellowship as a fully trained cardiac surgeon from McGill. It was the first time that we had taken on a trained cardiac surgeon. She was also the most driven of our fellows, wanting to simultaneously pursue a career as an astronaut, as well as a vascular surgeon. During Marlene's time, she became the most prolific of resident authors and was the first author of the division's only *New England Journal of Medicine* publication (Grenon, Gagnon, and Hsiang 2009).

Marlene's talents were recognized by other institutions; after the fellowship, she was recruited to UCSF where she is associate professor of surgery. Although the idea of being an astronaut may have taken a back seat, she has pursued other interests and is currently involved in the business development of new medical start-up companies.

Dr. Pascal Rheaume (2008–2010)

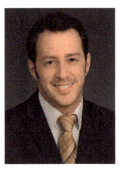

Dr. Pascal Rheaume (not the hockey player), was our third French Canadian fellow after Joel Gagnon and Marlene Grenon. Like Joel, he received his basic medical and general surgery training from Laval. And as with Joel, we were instructed by his chief, Dr. Yvan Douville, to "keep our mitts off him." I could not understand why, after the experience of losing a talent like Joel, they would send another outstanding (and unattached!) talent and risk him being seconded to the West. Fortunately for Laval and Pascal, the forces of Eros were unsuccessful, and he returned to Laval after his fellowship. Pascal is currently at the Hopital St-Francois D'Assise, Quebec City, QC.

Dr. Musaad Alghamdi (2008–2010)

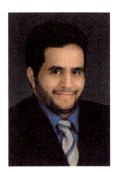 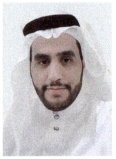

Dr. Musaad Alghamdi was our last graduate from Saudi Arabia; he completed his vascular surgery training in 2010. He spent an additional year doing interventional and endovascular surgery. After returning to Saudi Arabia, he was appointed to the academic staff at King Khalid University, where he is currently an assistant professor. He is also a consultant vascular surgeon at the Asir Central Hospital. He expressed his appreciation:

"Thanks (to) what I learned and mastered during my training in Vancouver, I (am) able to practice vascular and interventional radiology with confidence and dedication, especially since I found one of the graduates of Vancouver working in the same hospital, Dr. Muhammad Assiri. The harmony in the work with the spirit of one team became an example among other medical departments, and this also was what I saw and learned from my staff in Vancouver."

Dr. Matthew Robinson (2010–2012)

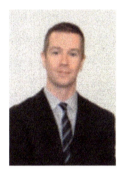

Dr. Matt Robinson graduated from the University of Manitoba before coming out west to start a pediatric residency at UBC. It was in his first year of pediatrics that he realized he preferred pediatric general surgery over pediatrics and transferred to the general surgery program. Soon after, he also discovered he enjoyed looking after patients at the other end of the age spectrum, and with that knowledge entered the vascular fellowship. He was a star fellow and would frequently challenge the surgeons regarding their decisions. After the fellowship, Matt settled in Victoria where he remains today, practising at Royal Jubilee Hospital. During his off-time, he may be found windsurfing in the Turks and Caicos.

Dr. Nadra Ginting (2010–2012)

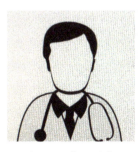

Dr. Nadra Ginting received her MD from the University of Toronto. She and Matt Robinson were in the same cohort for the 2010–12 class. After the vascular fellowship, she practised briefly in Abbotsford before relocating to join Matt at the Royal Jubilee Hospital in Victoria. Nadra, or "Nads" to her friends, is an avid frisbee player.

Dr. Daniel Kopac (2011–2013)

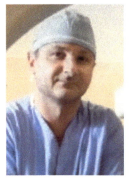

Dr. Dan Kopac graduated from the University of Alberta and completed his general surgery training there before coming to UBC for his vascular fellowship. Prior to medical school, Dan loved organic chemistry and stunned us with his knowledge of the unpronounceable new oral anticoagulants. After his fellowship, Dan settled in Richmond, BC where he works with Gord Houston.

Dr. Steven Johnson (2013–2015)

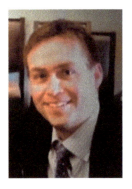

Dr. Steve Johnson was our last vascular surgery fellow. He completed his medical school at the University of Ottawa before coming west for general surgery training at the University of Calgary. After completing the vascular fellowship, he settled in Kamloops, BC, where he practices with Aristotle Azad. Steven was a deadly debater and became the obvious UBC banner-bearer for the Pacific Northwest vascular meetings, where the surgeons would be entertained with lively debates between residents of different programs.

Dr. Virginia Gunn (2015)

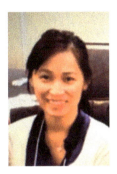

Our first graduate from the new Vascular Surgery residency, Dr. Virginia Gunn, a Vancouverite, graduated from the University of Western Ontario before returning to UBC for general surgery training. As a first-year resident in general surgery, she assisted Tony Salvian with a ruptured AAA. That was the motivation she needed to change to vascular surgery when the option became available. After completing the residency, Virginia spent time as a locum vascular surgeon at Royal Columbian Hospital before assuming a full-time position at the Grey Nuns Hospital in Edmonton, AB, along with two of our former fellows, Rob Turnbull and Gerrit Winkelaar. Being a Vancouverite and a foodie, when she is not on-call, Virginia makes frequent weekend trips home to see her family and enjoy the ethnic cuisine.

Dr. Kyle Arsenault (2019)

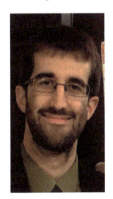

Dr. Kyle Arsenault graduated from McMaster University and entered the residency in 2014. After completion, he returned to Ontario where he now practices at the Peterborough Regional Health Centre.

Kyle was the fittest resident in the program, and enjoyed running everywhere. During his residency, Kyle married a future obstetrician and had a son. Reportedly, he has Kyle's running legs, so a future runner is expected in the family.

Dr. Jennifer Culig (2019)

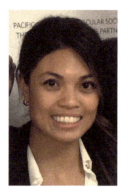

Dr. Jennifer Culig graduated from the University of Saskatchewan and was the second Saskatchewan graduate in the residency after Jon Misskey. During her time as a resident, Jen was fearless, and was part of a resident exchange program with the National University of Columbia in Bogota, Columbia. Her supervisor, Dr. Alberto Munoz, is the world authority on high-altitude-induced carotid body tumours, and Jen was part of his research team when she was in Bogota. She learned to speak Spanish during her time there, and when she returned to Vancouver, gave a fascinating round on living in Bogota, a bustling city of ten million people almost seven thousand feet above sea level. After completing the residency, Jen returned to Saskatchewan where she works in the "other" St. Paul's Hospital—in Saskatoon.

Dr. Gary Yang (2020)

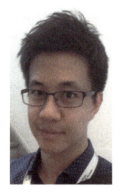

Dr. Gary Yang is the most recent graduate of our program. He recalls coming to Canada with his family as immigrants and describes his path to vascular surgery:

"I was born as Yang Kai-Yuan in Taiwan and grew up in the Banqiao District with my parents, James and Maggie, and my brother Kevin. Shortly after my tenth birthday, we immigrated to Burnaby, BC. Moving to North America was what any able Chinese parents would do for their children back in the 1990s. *Gary* was the English name given to me by my English tutor, Gary—not exactly a creative fellow. Fitting into a new culture proved difficult. French as a third language at Brantford Elementary was comical when my English was limited to *yes, no,* and my own name, which I spelled wrong on more than one occasion.

Fast forward to the final year of my bachelor's degree in Physiology; I worked closely with my research supervisor, Dr. Kenny Kwok. It had been a passion and goal for me to pursue a career in education. My time spent on rodent surgeries further solidified my plan to pursue an academic career. I met Dr. Tim Kieffer, already a world-renowned researcher in diabetes. Together, Kenny and Tim co-supervised my PhD to develop a new murine *in situ* perfusion model to better elucidate the signalling pathways of gastric and pancreatic hormones and their potential significance in diabetes. This was perhaps when my vascular surgery training began.

Near the end of my PhD training, I studied abroad at the University of Warwick in the UK. It was in the small town of Coventry where I made the decision to go to medical school in order to become a clinician scientist, and continue my work in diabetes. But, in Canada, to pursue a career in endocrinology you have to go to Toronto, the site where insulin was discovered.

I was assigned to the inaugural class at the Mississauga Academy of Medicine, but I also spent time at the Banting and Best Research Centre. There I met Dr. David Cherney, an academic nephrologist with a research interest in type 1 diabetes mellitus. David took me under his wing and allowed me to continue my academic pursuits. On paper, I was on a clear path toward endocrinology. However, I missed working with my hands, perhaps reminiscing about the days operating on rodent aortas.

My first clerkship rotation in vascular surgery was at the Mississauga Hospital, where I met Dr. Ahmed Kayssi, an inspiring general surgery resident with plans of pursuing a vascular surgery fellowship. Ahmed shared his passion and enthusiasm about becoming an academic vascular surgeon. By the end of the rotation, I also shared Ahmed's dream. The long pursuit toward endocrinology thus came to a halt. But, knowing that vascular surgeons deal with diabetics was a reasonable compromise.

Returning to Vancouver and UBC certainly was nostalgic. I was quickly greeted by York Hsiang, who soon became my new mentor and pillar. Working closely with York, I found myself back at the UBC animal facility performing surgeries on rat carotid arteries. We also worked together in organizing the annual BC Vascular Day meetings to bring together health care workers across the province. Now as a young staff member, I am fortunate to have York as a mentor, adviser, and friend.

Dave Taylor is the backbone of UBC Vascular Surgery. His presence demands attention—not out of fear, but out of respect. However, he also has a keen sense of humour. This was on full display when he summarized my "Yang Manoeuvres:"

1. *Don't pass the suture.* After tying down the heel of an end-to-side anastomosis, one of the sutures must be passed underneath the knot to the other side. Failure to do so will generate deep shame, as I learned the hard way. Despite my insistence that I had done so, it is hard to argue against the end result of a Prolene suture running across the hood of the graft. Nothing makes you want to hide in the corner more than a staff member cutting out your anastomosis.

2. *The 360 twist.* Twisting a tunnelled bypass is a feared complication of all vascular surgeons. However, twisting an *in situ* vein graft by 360 degrees takes intentional effort. The end result is a water hammer pulse, even though the blue dots are technically still on top. How this happened in my hands remains an unsolved mystery—I am known to surprise people.

3. *Butterfingers.* Dave Taylor claims that this has never happened before in his operating room, but I know this is not true after a conversation with an alumnus who shall remain nameless. After preparing a good-sized saphenous vein to patch an extensive femoral endarterectomy, the artery clamp along with the vein succumbed to gravity. What was probably half a second felt like an eternity. "Did that just happen?" asked the scrub nurse, breaking the silence. Fortunately, we were able to harvest more vein.

Why do these mishaps only happen in Dave's OR? Perhaps he is the only one that keeps track with periodic reminders. However, he is also one of the few that will laugh with you about it afterwards.

While many reminisce about the midnight rupture or the twelve-hour bypass, the most memorable events in residency often happen outside the hospital. Social events allowed us to remove our labels and sit as equals. Even if it was at the house of the Godfather, Tony Salvian. (How did he get that name, you ask? I fear I have already disclosed too much.) Sometimes it also provided the opportunity to best the mentors—or so I thought. Bubble ball soccer involves everyone wearing a giant inflatable bouncy bubble and has very little to do with soccer. It is a game of tackling and shoulder checking, unless you are going up against the 6'4" Jon Misskey or the more grounded Keith Baxter. Nothing says *Welcome to the division!* better than whiplash and "Stay down!"

Halfway through my residency training, Jerry Chen took over as the program director. The first resident retreat he organized was a nice short hike in Squamish. As it turns out, *nice* is subjective and *short* is a lie. The four-hour hike up the appropriately named Sea to Summit Trail, where a sane person will take a gondola, was really a way for Jerry to say that I still have a long way to go to become the best Taiwanese vascular surgeon in Canada, inside and outside of the OR.

In my third year of residency, the UBC Vascular program found itself in a unique situation with four senior residents. Perhaps for the first, and likely the last time, the program had a surplus of residents. Keith Baxter reached out to satellite sites to enrich the training experience. I was fortunate to be one of the first vascular trainees to step into the Okanagan. I had heard tales from Ahmed back in medical school about the utopic practice in Kelowna where four friends shared a practice. The training I received from Drs. Jeremy Harris, Kirk Lawlor, Stephen Mostowy, and Jeff Pasenau forged the rest of my development into a vascular surgeon. More importantly, without reservation, they each invited me into their homes, their families, and their lives. I am proud to call them my friends and my new partners. Perhaps it was the hospitality, the friendly smiles, or the sweet Rieslings, but when they offered me to join their practice, I accepted without hesitation—I would have been a fool not to."

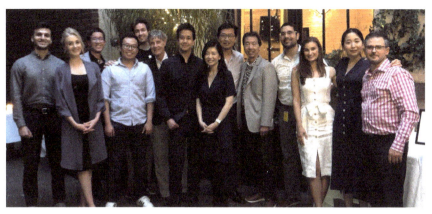

Gary Yang's graduation dinner. Left to right: Abdalla Butt (R), Alexa Mordhorst (R), Adrian Fung (R), Bill Huang (R), Jon Misskey, Jock Reid, Gary Yang, Chongya Yang, Jerry Chen, YNH, Gautamn Sarwal (R), Eva Angelopoulos, Sally Choi (R), Joel Gagnon. (R) = Resident. c. 2020.

PART SEVEN

THE CONSTANT: ROSALINE CHUNG

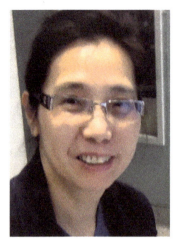

"Hey Roz, can you help me?" came the cry from the nurse across the hall. "I need to get the man up so I can make his bed." As always, Roz was a willing helper. But, today, she was thanked in the most unceremonious way. The man was agitated, and thinking there was a nearby toilet, he let loose a steady stream of yellow fluid all over Roz. "Aargh!" exclaimed both Roz and the nurse. Although it was nasty, it was just another day for Roz at VGH.

For forty-one years, Rosaline ("Roz") Chung served as the Vascular Surgery unit clerk from its origin in the Heather Pavilion, all the way to the Jim Pattison Tower. But it was never supposed to be like this. She was a student nurse from Hong Kong when her family immigrated to Canada. With her training only partially completed, she had planned on completing her RN training at VGH. Instead, while still a student nurse, a unit clerk position became available when the latest clerk decided to quit. "Roz," said Miss Harrison, the Vascular Surgery head nurse, "fill in as the unit clerk until I can find a replacement." Having never trained to work as a unit clerk, Roz used her nursing background to organize how she thought the work of a unit clerk should be done. In fact, she filled in so well that when a new clerk was finally recruited, nobody wanted to surrender Roz.

With her organizational abilities and "BS detector," Roz quickly became the glue that held the ward together through changes in management, nurses, residents, and students. Doctors were persuaded to write clear and legible orders, nurses were instructed to undertake the doctors' orders, escorts were scheduled to take patients for tests and to the OR, needed inventory was ordered before supplies ran out, and pads of different requisitions were arranged in sensible categories. These were the unwritten Rules of Roz. Even though she had no formal training as a unit clerk, her methods were so efficient she became an educator for many unit clerks throughout the hospital. If you wanted to know anything about anybody on the ward, just ask Roz. Those who feared her knew they had to get on her good side in order to get anything done. The surgeons loved her, trusting her to look after their patients and their personal lives, from car keys to other personal effects.

But the grind of working in a large teaching hospital is like being subjected to Chinese water torture. At first the drips are irritating but tolerable. Then the drops become noticeably more frequent and progressively more annoying until your head feels like exploding with each one. Like many good people, the constant bickering with management led to Roz taking "early" retirement after forty-one years. However, as a workaholic, not working as a hospital unit clerk did not mean she would actually retire. Throughout her tenure at VGH, Roz also ran her own private tutoring company: Brainchild. And when on holidays each summer, she worked at the Pacific National Exhibition.

So, after leaving VGH, Roz worked for a short time as a secretary for well-known liver transplant surgeon, Dr. Charles "Buzz" Scudamore. That position was temporary and when Buzz's secretary came back from maternity leave, I had the good fortune of being able to recruit Roz to be my medical office assistant (MOA). Despite having no MOA training and not knowing how to type, she filled in admirably. For the last twelve years, I have received numerous compliments about my MOA: she answers the phone after three rings, doesn't put patients on hold, and is there first thing in the morning—at half past six in the morning. You could say that Roz has been the glue keeping my office together.

Epilogue

Into the Unknown

Vancouver is a hockey town and the Canucks are king. The Canucks have been in the NHL since 1970 and have come close to winning the Stanley Cup three times, but have never won. Why other newer teams have been more successful than the hapless Canucks is open to speculation. Could it be that the players, coaches, or both, become distracted from their primary purpose when they come to Vancouver with its natural beauty? To some Vancouverites, when former Canuck coach Mike Keenan addressed their top player, Trevor Linden, with "Trevor, you're a good player, but don't you want to be a great player?" it was perceived as crossing a line. But what if Keenan was speaking the truth? And what if there is a trickle-down effect in Vancouver that permeates sports, business, and academia?

For the forty years since its origin, the VGH Vascular Surgery Division has grown, with more faculty, teaching programs, research, and outreach into the national and international communities of vascular surgeons. It continues with its excellent training program for students and residents. This makes it a good division. It has at times been a great division, with the daring and tenacity to push new boundaries in clinical practices and research innovations. But, will it be able to exceed its past achievements in the next forty years, let alone maintain its current position? There are many headwinds from both the university and the hospital, but headwinds, obstructions, and the like have always existed. They are challenges that need to be viewed as such and dealt with.

Each vascular surgery division is different. The differences are almost always due to factors that involve people: personalities, events, struggles, outcomes, and consequences. Like many, we have won as many struggles as we have lost. For the struggles we won, we need to review how we achieved success when the outlook was uncertain. For the struggles we lost, we need to review the reasons why we thought our position was just, and the choices that were made, to avoid making the same mistake again. Recognizing errors and rectifying them is always difficult, since none of us are good at apologizing. There will be always be future challenges whether obvious or opaque, and we need to be ready. After all, we are vascular surgeons—what we do is to preserve life and function. Planning is our strength and we lead with strength.

Lumen accipe et imperti. Accept the light and pass it on.

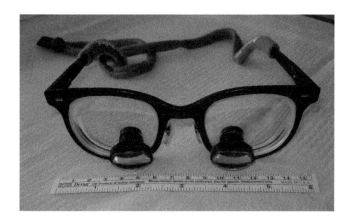

Appendix A

WHAT THEY NEVER TAUGHT ME

IN MEDICAL SCHOOL

CONTENTS

1. Forward
2. What is Vascular Surgery?
3. Why You Should Choose a Rotation in Vascular Surgery
4. Problems with Medical School Education (applied to the lower extremity)
5. Getting on the Right Side of People
   a. In the Operating Room
   b. On the Ward
6. Collecting Evidence
   a. History Taking
      i. Leg Pain
      ii. Swelling
      iii. What is the Most Important *P*?
   b. Use of Doppler and ABI
7. How to Give a Presentation
8. How to Request a Reference Letter

1. Forward

There are so many thoughts about your career, like how you ended up with the career you chose, to the things you saw, and the people you met. All of us though, acquire a body of knowledge that is unique through all of these experiences, and how we respond to them. Good or bad, these choices become part of our body of knowledge. So, when confronted with a similar episode, we seemingly know what to do. This knowledge is not found in traditional medical school or residency training. Each physician carries with them the sum experience of their collective thoughts and experiences, and it is a shame that younger physicians have to relearn it in the most fundamental state—usually under duress, which always leaves an indelible impression. So, rather than leave it to the novice to discover, the aim of this appendix for medical students is to speed up the learning curve, emphasizing what really is important, and how to avoid problems. It is my hope that other physicians may choose to use the same format and create their own lasting experiences.

2. What is Vascular Surgery?

Vascular surgery is the surgical specialty of treating diseases of the blood vessels, with the exception of those in the brain or in the heart. Hence, arteries and veins (as well as lymphatics), large and small, are the domain of vascular surgeons. Unlike most other specialties (with the exception of ophthalmology and ENT) in Canada, there is no medical counterpart to vascular surgery, like cardiology and cardiac surgery. In the United States and Europe, however, there is the specialty of Vascular Medicine, which serves as a medical counterpart. Hence, vascular surgeons in Canada also treat vascular diseases medically.

Vascular surgery is a new specialty, having formally acquired specialty status in the early 1980s. It used to be a subspecialty of general surgery, meaning that having endured a general surgery residency, you needed to do an extra two years as a vascular surgery fellow. That program (five years of general surgery residency plus two years of vascular fellowship) continues in some centres in the United States, but in Canada, vascular surgery became a direct entry program from medical school in 2012. Being able to match directly into vascular surgery means shortening your training by two years, although you will not have the designation of being a double fellow in general and vascular surgery.

Although the subspecialty is narrow, the diseases covered are broad. The most common venous problem is varicose veins, an age-related condition that occurs in up to 50 percent of the population. On the other hand, more serious arterial problems, such as aneurysms and peripheral arterial disease, occur in up to 10 percent of the elderly population. Because of the time-limited exposure you have in medical school, only the most serious diseases, such as AAAs and other arterial diseases, are formally taught, whereas the most common problems, such as varicose veins, are barely mentioned. Recognizing that most medical students become primary care physicians, it is imperative to learn on your own about the most common diseases that will fill your practice on a daily basis.

As a result of not having a medical counterpart and the broad training required, vascular surgeons need to provide a continuous spectrum of care from diagnosis, including ultrasound and angiographic imaging, to all interventional procedures (endovascular and surgical) as well as perform wound care and amputations of the diseased limb. This "one stop care" simplifies the main care provider for the patient, and is rewarding for the surgeon.

3. Why You Should Choose a Rotation in Vascular Surgery

No matter where your interests lie, you should consider doing a rotation in vascular surgery. If your interest is in medicine, then being on a vascular surgery ward is where you will find the "best" patients. These male and female patients are all "wrecks" with the most advanced physical signs. Frequently, internists troll our wards for patients to teach. Bruits, murmurs, malnutrition, fluid balance challenges, crepitations and edema—vascular patients have it all. This is because advanced vascular diseases do not respond to medical treatment. So, one of the fundamental differences of this specialty compared to others is that all patients who require urgent vascular surgery because of advanced ischemia or enormous aneurysms are rarely turned down unless, of course, they are palliative patients. Consequently, the breadth of medical illnesses, such as advanced complicated diabetes, renal failure (including the need for dialysis), coronary artery disease, chronic lung diseases, etc., can all be found in vascular surgery patients.

On the other hand, if your interest is in surgery, then there is no finer rotation for you. As one of my colleagues puts it, vascular surgeons are the "firefighters of the operating room," putting out fires (i.e., stopping bleeding) when they occur! Operating all over the body except in the brain and in the heart, the procedures vary from the fine and delicate, for example, using sutures the thickness of a hair, to the big and bulky procedures, such as amputation.

Even medical students interested in psychiatry will find it worthwhile, as post-op confusion and alcohol withdrawal occurs in at least half of our patients! As a medical student, you want to see lots of things and encounter difficult pathologies in the most challenging patients. Vascular surgery will give you that.

4. Problems with Medical School Education (applied to the lower extremity)

During the three to four years of medical school education, the poor medical student has to master a completely new language, memorize an immense number of facts, and acquire basic scientific understanding. And, all of this knowledge has to be at one's fingertips any time of day or night.

On top of that, medical students are usually chosen based not only on their academic abilities but also on their "humanness." Applicants who are only smart and work hard will no longer suffice. Instead, medical schools seek supermen and superwomen to replace the current generation of physicians. Having abilities and experiences outside of medicine, such as being athletic, interested in the arts, and volunteering in many activities, are all perceived to make one a superior physician. In reality, how this criterion is superior to previous selection criteria is completely unknown. What is known is that the discipline of medicine is so broad it can accommodate any qualified student's personality. For instance, you could choose anything from specialties that have tremendous patient exposure to specialties where you will never meet any patients (at least not live ones). After teaching many medical students, the only useful requirements that stick out to me in selecting medical students are for them to be hard working, gifted with a fantastic memory, and have the ability to function at full capacity with minimal sleep. Tired is what you will be as a medical student and later a physician, but no admission committee will evaluate applicants when they are sleep deprived.

Consequently, with such a diverse group, and the need for them to acquire the skills to be a physician, medical school education is, essentially, about pigeon-holing information. Many medical school educators may disagree with this concept, as will students in their first or second year, when everything they learn is so new and interesting. Broadening medical students' concept of the whole patient is the basis of problem-based learning where educators serve as facilitators and allow students to delve into discussions of their own. While good for natural inquisitiveness, it does not help the student prepare for the next step. Residency requires the new physician to be able to compile a thorough history, perform a comprehensive examination, develop a working diagnosis, initiate investigations, and write up the findings all within twenty minutes. Thus, to go from a mass of unstructured facts to a focused plan requires learning the art and language of medicine in a structured fashion.

During medical school however, the predominant teachers are specialists. These specialist physician educators tend to cram many facts, anecdotes, and pictures into their talks to emphasize the importance of their specialty. Consequently, with so many available facts to learn, who will emphasize what is really important?

The teaching of the lower extremity is an example of a deficient area of medical school education. Usually, the back, chest, abdominal cavities, upper extremity, and certain systems such as cardiovascular are well taught, primarily because of the time allotted to these areas. By the time the lower extremities need to be taught, it is usually at the end of an exhaustive educational block. Is it any wonder that most physicians know nothing about feet, posture, and mobility? Yet, more and more studies recognize the beneficial effects of walking, from weight control to good cardiovascular and mental health. To walk is to live.

5. Getting on the Right Side of People

A. IN THE OPERATING ROOM

For any new trainee, what separates surgery from other disciplines is the operating room. Affectionately known as the operating theatre, OR, or various other names in different parts of the world, this is an exciting place of controlled violence and the miracle of modern anesthesia.

To most surgeons and OR staff, having medical students is a hindrance. To get on the good side of nurses, the minimum you need to know is OR etiquette and sterility. In the OR, everybody dresses in the same coloured scrubs, hats, and masks, and nobody can tell whether you are a physician or nurse, let alone a medical, nursing, or other type of student. Since the key to avoiding conflict is good communication, let the OR staff know who you are, what level you are at, and what your glove size is, if you are going to scrub. If you are not good at certain things, let people know. Don't try to conceal anything. Apart from fainting and falling into the wound, the next worst thing to do is to contaminate the sterile field or grab instruments from the scrub nurse's back table.

Once scrubbed, it is always okay to ask questions. There is usually a steady banter throughout the case, often at the opening and closing of the case. To keep the students and residents involved in the case, the surgeon usually quizzes them on anatomy, pathology, or patient management. Often times, "pimping" (the affectionate term for asking difficult questions) is done in a reverse hierarchical fashion with the most junior medical student getting the question first, and if they can't answer it, then the question is passed up the "food chain" to the next level student or resident. To avoid being pimped on continuously, the astute medical student should ask all the questions to minimize pimping time. Moments of complete silence usually reflect a critical stage of the procedure. During these times, questions and jokes should be avoided.

The typical task that a medical student may be given is to do something simple such as cut sutures, tie a knot, or staple or sew skin. Whenever you are given a new task that you have not done before, ask the surgeon to show you *how they would do it*. For instance, if your task is to cut the sutures, always ask the surgeon how they want the sutures cut (hence the usual medical student response of "too long or too short"). If you really don't know, then ask. (Show me a medical student who only doubles my work, and I will kiss their feet!) I have no expectations as to what a medical student can do, so I always assume they are complete novices at everything.

B. ON THE WARD

There's a reason why medical students are frequently considered "door jams"—their main role is to open the doors for all the other medical staff. No matter how much you think you know, there is always somebody who knows more. And this applies when dealing with nurses, clerks, and even orderlies at times. They have spent years doing the same job and have seen so much more than you have during your brief foray on the wards. Defer to them, and they will teach you all kinds of proper and efficient ways of doing simple tasks like changing dressings and removing sutures and drains, and how to do more technical tasks such as removing chest tubes and tracheostomies.

Besides, these folks can also make your life difficult if they perceive you need to be "brought down a few rungs." Ridiculous (to you) calls in the middle of the night because of patients with chest pain, with fever, who can't pee, who can't stop peeing, who can't sleep (that makes two of you!) make up a never-ending cycle of the nurses testing your knowledge, team spirit, and organizational abilities (you should have done an eleven o'clock evening round to tidy up the loose ends). In medicine, everybody needs to be treated properly, not just the patient.

6. Collecting Evidence

There are two major problems with medical student education: the lack of understanding of terms both in scientific and lay usage, and the weighting of historical or physical findings. Let me illustrate. When you refer to the *circulation*, what do you mean? How do you measure circulation? As you may recall, circulation refers to the movement of blood from the heart through the arteries to every part of the body and returning via the veins to the heart. So, for circulation to exist, you need a beating heart, an artery, and a vein as the minimum requirement. But, how do you measure this? Even worse, when a patient says they "have something wrong with their circulation," what do they mean and how do you investigate this?

The logical response is to assess the arterial inflow and venous return separately, and possibly the lymphatic function, to get an idea if there is a problem with the arteries, veins, or lymphatics. But the term *circulation* is something we all know vaguely about. However, there is not one measurement we use to measure its viability or sickness.

Similarly, how do you measure metabolism, immunity, and the like? Again, we have a vague idea what these are, but there is no single measurement for any of these terms. So, a better definition of commonly used terms needs to be stressed both by physicians and lay people.

The other problem with medical education is the lack of emphasizing the importance of weighting the information you collect (e.g., history, physical signs) or even the tests you order when making a diagnosis. As an example, consider the signs we stress to medical students when examining the foot using the Inspection, Palpation, and Auscultation method (there is no Percussion used when examining the foot).

For inspection, one can comment on the colour of the foot and whether there are any gross features such as the shape, missing digits, odour, and swelling. In reality, the value of these features is not equal. Gross things such as loss of digits, completely black toes, and ulcers are really important because they signify gangrenous changes—a dangerous situation for the patient because it usually indicates advanced ischemia and the likelihood of needing amputation of the toe or foot. The general colour, on the other hand—pale, blue, or purple, is not that important because the colour of the foot is determined by blood vessels of the skin, both the arteries and the veins. There may be an underlying problem with the major blood vessels or there could be only a skin blood flow issue such as vasoconstriction. Similarly, a blue or purple foot could be something very sinister, such as DVT, or extremely benign, such as venous congestion from sitting too long.

Astute students may recognize this as placing probabilities around certain features to diagnose an underlying condition. Terms such as *sensitivity*, *specificity*, and *predictive values* are the basis of clinical epidemiology and use simple mathematics to make better estimates for the likelihood of certain conditions.

Instead, we promote useless facts such as the diagnostic value of a named test to diagnose conditions. Consider this worthless example that all medical students have memorized: Homer's sign: calf pain with dorsiflexion of the foot may indicate DVT. The diagnostic value of Homer's sign is only 50 percent, so it is no better than a guess. Instead of perpetuating useless tests and reasoning, medical school should emphasize key features that would rapidly rule a disease in or out. For instance, in the situation of a suspected DVT, there are no infallible clinical features and the early recommendation of ultrasound is the best test to rapidly prove or disprove the condition.

A.   History Taking

As with most areas of medicine, a good history will usually lead you to the right diagnosis. There are, however, certain questions that, when asked, point to a certain diagnosis. Some medical students may recognize this as "increasing the pre-test likelihood" to determine a certain diagnosis. Unfortunately, most medical students use long lists of questions and apply equal weight to the answers. During the history, the aim is to not only achieve the correct diagnosis, but also to determine the severity of a patient's symptoms in order to determine how quickly treatment needs to be initiated.

i. Leg Pain

To highlight this, I have chosen leg pain and swelling as the most common symptoms encountered in vascular surgery. Most commonly, leg pain may be due to problems associated with muscles, joints, or nerves. The leg anatomically describes the calf, so the astute medical student needs to determine which part of the leg the patient is referring to. Joint pain always occurs in joints and is never due to arterial insufficiency. Apart from fatigue as a result of over exercising, calf or thigh muscular pain is due to either arterial insufficiency or related to neuropathy. This is the basis of arteriogenic or neurogenic claudication.

The most discerning questions to distinguish these two conditions relate to the onset of symptoms, aggravating factors, and relieving factors. For instance, arterial insufficiency does not occur when there is a postural change such as when a patient stands up. It is only caused by exercise (unless, of course, the patient has pain all the time—a more severe condition known as *rest pain*). Since the calf muscle is the most oxygen-dependent muscle used during walking, pain is invariably felt in the calf. Also, as the gastrocnemius muscles are the most important calf muscles for walking, the pain is usually noted in the posterior calf. The walking distance is invariably reproducible, meaning the patient can only walk the same distance each time before needing to stop. Once the patient stops walking, the pain is relieved. It is highly unusual for it to be associated with numbness (unless again, if associated with more advanced ischemia such as rest pain).

On the other hand, the quality of the pain is unimportant. People have different pain thresholds; some people describe their pain as heaviness, whereas others describe it as a sharp or dull sensation.

So, the most important questions (and suggestive answers) to enquire for peripheral arterial disease are:

- Where is the pain? (posterior calf, may be thigh or buttock depending on the level of occlusion)
- How far can you walk? (fixed distance) Each time? (yes, each time)
- Is it improved with rest? (yes)

Conversely, important negative questions are:

- Does the pain occur when you first stand up? (no)
- Does the pain get better with exercise? (no)
- Does the pain spread into the lower back? (no)

ii. Swelling

The approach to swelling is similar. Swelling may be due to excess water or lymph. The astute medical student will recognize this as an exudate or transudate—the distinguishing clinical feature is whether they have pitting edema or not on physical examination. There are systemic and local causes of both. Limiting this discussion to local swelling, the key questions are related to the onset, one or both limbs, and the extent of the swelling (e.g., foot, leg or higher).

Swelling (edema) is a feature of venous conditions and not arterial. Usually, for the latter, the problem is that there is not enough blood reaching the extremity rather than having too much blood that cannot return to the heart. A venous problem may be related to venous reflux (e.g., varicose veins or deep venous insufficiency) or venous obstruction (e.g., DVT). In this case, the edema is pitting. Non-pitting edema is due to a lymphatic problem until proven otherwise. The only rare time when swelling can be due to arterial insufficiency is when the ischemia is so advanced that the patient has to sleep in an upright position. In this position, gravity aids blood flow, so the patient's pain is improved (this is also a feature of rest pain). When subjected to gravity (i.e., the legs are kept in a dependent position) for an extended time, lower extremity edema will occur. This is much like ankle swelling after a long plane flight.

Local swelling is almost always a venous problem. Acutely, one needs to rule out DVT. Chronically, it is often related to venous reflux of the superficial or deep system. Thus, the important questions to ask are:

- Where is the swelling? (foot, leg, or higher)
- One or both legs?
- Is it associated with a colour change or anything else?

iii. What is the Most Important P?

Through rote memorization, medical students all know of the six "*p*"s that indicate acute arterial ischemia: **p**ain, **p**allor, **p**hrygidity or **p**oikilothermia (meaning cold!), **p**ulselessness, **p**aresthesia, and **p**aralysis. But, do you need all six to have acute arterial ischemia? What if you only have four or five "*p*"s?

The dilemma really occurs when you are confronted with a patient whom you think may have this condition. What do you do? Most likely you will call your immediate superior, either a resident or consultant. They will only ask you one question, "Can they move the limb?" All they are interested in is whether there is paralysis or not! But, how do you test for that? In the calf, the most oxygen sensitive muscle compartment is the anterior compartment which is responsible for dorsiflexion of the ankle. Can they move the limb means: "Can they actively dorsiflex the ankle?"

Why would they only be interested in this movement alone? The reason is that paralysis (excluding any other neurologic cause) indicates insufficient blood flow to the muscle. In that situation there is a limited window to revascularize the ischemic muscle before irreversible muscle necrosis sets in. The usual window is six hours from the onset of paralysis. This means that the presence of paralysis is a surgical emergency and needs immediate revascularization.

So, again, each of the six "p"s do not have equal weight. They may all indicate some degree of ischemia, but it is the presence of paralysis that is most important. None of the other "p"s mandate immediate surgery.

B.   USE OF DOPPLER AND ABI

When it comes to measuring the adequacy of arterial flow, there is a lot of emphasis placed on palpating for pulses, including the range of strength of pulses from very weak to bounding. As our abilities to perceive subtle differences using our hands is limited, the most objective method of measuring pulses is not with our hands, but with Doppler. The use of Doppler to measure arterial flow is far superior to palpating for pulses as it has greater sensitivity (ability to measure arterial flow at a lower blood pressure) and is far more reliable.

The ankle-brachial index (ABI) is a ratio of the systolic blood pressures of the ankle to the arm. When there is a slight discrepancy between the arm blood pressures, the higher arm blood pressure is used as the reference. If there is a wide difference between the arm pressures, then again you will use the higher arm blood pressure, but you may have also discovered a subclavian artery stenosis or occlusion that is causing the lower arm blood pressure.

At the level of the ankle, blood pressure is measured from the dorsalis pedis and posterior tibial arteries. By convention, we choose the higher ABI of the two pedal arteries as indicative of the patient's ABI. Readers are directed to review the video we made specifically for this.[60]

7. How to Give a Presentation

One of the requirements of being a resident and possibly after residency is to give a presentation. So, it's a good idea to accept the challenge of presenting. There are many advantages and no disadvantages. First, for a while you may appear as the key resource person on the topic since you would have read the most recently published articles about it. Second, you can control the discussion by asking questions of other students, residents, and staff during the presentation. Doing so deflects questions away from you and demonstrates that you are engaging the audience. Third, with each presentation you will learn things about what you did right and where you could improve on. So, try and pick a topic you know nothing about. By the time you have done several presentations they will start to become easier and who knows, maybe you will have the opportunity of presenting to a larger audience at a major conference. These are the best opportunities since you will be exposing yourself to all the right people who may be making decisions about your future.

A few suggestions about presentations:

- Know your audience. Find out who you are talking to, then tailor your talk for the audience. Your first few slides will be simple introductory or refresher slides, and then you can slowly delve into the topic more deeply. If you are uncertain of the topic, then always start generally before making it more technical.

- Continued reinforcement is key. After your introductory slide, you may want to explain what you are going to talk about, then talk about it, and finally talk about what you just talked about, as part of the conclusion or summary.

- Less is more. Limit the number of words and sentences on your slide. You want the audience to listen to you rather than read what you have written. There are several suggested ranges, such as no more than five sentences per slide, and no more than five words per sentence. Make it what you need, but remember the KISS principle: Keep it simple, stupid!

- Use large fonts. The worst thing is to have a gazillion tiny words and no pictures. By using fewer words and sentences, you can enlarge the font so that anybody in the back row can read it comfortably.

- Rehearse to stay within the allotted time and have some time at the end for questions. If you have a buddy who is going to your talk, plant one or two questions for your buddy to ask to avoid embarrassing long pauses at the end.

- Remember that your talk should be both educational and entertaining. It helps to start off with a joke or have a short video clip during the presentation.

- It's not the fancy artwork on the slides but the content of what you are delivering that will make the most impact. Sometimes the best slides are the simplest. The most effective way to deliver information is by using open ended questions.

- Lastly, make sure you know how the microphone and slide advancer work before you start.

8. How to Request a Reference Letter

Unfortunately, since Canadian medical schools no longer issue letter grades or marks, there is no objective measurement of a medical student's abilities. While this may be fine for some, it creates considerable havoc when it comes to selecting students directly from medical school. The only way assessors can determine whether they would be interested in a particular medical student for their program is by the reference letter. The only other way of assessing a medical student may be via a short interview, but you need to get invited to the interview first, as most programs do not interview all the potential candidates. Medical students are also asked to write a personal testimony on why they want to be matched to a specific program, but assessors take very little notice of this. So, the reference letter becomes vitally important.

For the reference letter, one needs to be selective and assertive. When asking for a letter of reference, the key things to remember are:

- How many letters do you need? Typically, three reference letters are required. You could send more, but they may not be read. Since the reference letter is about the only objective information available about you, each reference letter needs to be *exemplary*. An average reference letter is a red flag that you were not an impressive student who did not make a lasting impression.
- Who will you get the reference letters from? The typical dilemma here is choosing between a consultant you have

worked with and knows you well, but may not have a particularly high-status title, or a consultant who has higher status whom you do not know well. Generally, a better letter will come from somebody you worked with who was impressed by you.

- Will they write a (good) reference letter? Here the distinction is a *good* letter. A busy consultant or professor receives up to a dozen requests for reference letters each year. Typically, there is a template they use. Reviewers can spot a generic reference letter. So, when requesting a letter, you need to tactfully ask if they are able to supply a *good* reference letter.

- When do you approach them for a reference letter? If you think a specialty like vascular surgery could be your chosen future career, then commit to that. Serious interest can be demonstrated by arranging most of your electives in that specialty. Also, try to identify early on who you should approach to write a good reference letter. When approaching the surgeon for a reference letter, do it <u>before</u> the end of the rotation. If you ask them one or two weeks later, they likely have long forgotten about you. When you approach them for a letter, do something atypical, e.g., request to meet them in person, bring them a thank you card, etc. Something that makes you stand out.

- Make it easy for them. Let them know what the letter needs to cover, when the deadline is, if it's a specialty-specific or generic letter, the dates you were on the service, and if there was a specific case that you learned a lot from. It is also a good time to send them a picture of yourself plus an up-to-date resume.

- Good luck!

Appendix B

WHAT THEY NEVER
TAUGHT ME IN RESIDENCY

CONTENTS

1. Forward

When I transitioned from an intern to a resident, my life became more complicated. There was now more responsibility to the senior residents and surgeons above me, and the medical students and interns below. I also had been out of the operating room for a long time before starting residency so whatever rudimentary surgical skills I had were completely forgotten.

What I discovered was that surgeons come in all stripes. There were some who were kind, had patience, and recognized your limitations. And then there were those who had no patience for novices like me. I learned from all of them. It took hours of practise to develop skills, even more time for observing, and most importantly, recording each surgeon's nuances and idiosyncrasies. I did not progress rapidly until I finally "got the hang of it": how to use instruments, the force needed to handle different tissues, and when we could go fast and when to be slow and meticulous. By the time I completed my training, I knew how to operate, who to operate on, and had a vague idea of who not to operate on. And yet, I had no idea that life as a surgeon also meant being a diplomat, a psychologist, an administrator, and a small business owner. The following is a collection of "pearls" for residents at all levels of training, and some guidance for a young surgeon as a business person.

2. What Makes a Good Resident?

I am old-fashioned. I know you can't judge residents using one-liners anymore. Now you need to describe them in terms of professional, scholar, educator, collaborator, teacher, advocate, etc. Or, whatever all that means. I do know, having once been a resident, and having trained dozens of residents, what makes a good one. A lot of it is common sense but there are some other aspects that may surprise you.

A good resident is not the person who jokes with the staff surgeon trying to figure out which side his or her bread is buttered on. A good resident first and foremost is a good doctor. So, a good surgical resident needs to know a lot about internal medicine. All those complications will come back and bite you. Because after all the laughter is done, "dying with a patent graft" is really not funny at all.

Dedicated, careful, considerate, hard-working: these adjectives describe almost all residents. However, there are certain features that make for an outstanding resident.

Regardless of the level of resident, an outstanding one is prepared, enthusiastic, and ready to learn. What separates surgery from other areas of medicine is the "legalized controlled violence." Patients willingly give up their bodies for us to operate on. To be given that privilege, we can't "botch" procedures, and thereby lose their trust. This means that when we operate, our full attention is on that patient in front of us. A simple concept, but difficult to grasp until you become the surgeon—when the expectations of the patient, their relatives, and the operating room staff all become your responsibility. So, the difference between being the resident and given the privilege to learn on the consultant's patients, and being the consultant, is the constant anguish over deciding on the correct operation, executing it beautifully, and having to relinquish that authority to a lesser surgeon, i.e., the resident.

The earliest distinguishing feature of an outstanding resident is a readiness to learn. True learning comes from preparation and dedicated practise. The outstanding resident will prepare him or herself by being in the operating room before the consultant, having placed all of the relevant images on the computer or viewing board, met, interviewed, and examined the patient, read about the patient's condition, and read about the proposed operation. An outstanding senior resident would have done all of the above, but will also have read about the alternative procedures.

Once the resident has prepared in this fashion, they are ready to learn. The education of the surgical procedure with the staff surgeon starts pre-operatively by reviewing the images; discussing the case, including peculiarities; describing which procedure will be done and why that procedure was chosen over others; and discussing the expected findings and anticipated difficulties, as well as solutions to problems or intraoperative surprises. Usually, the discussion will continue during the pre-op scrub and draping of the patient. These are all "golden moments" for teaching—moments that should not be missed.

The hardest thing to teach is that which is innate and therefore, not teachable. A negative attitude is impossible to correct. Adjectives commonly used to describe a poor attitude are: *lazy, easily bored, uninterested, poorly prepared, rigid,* etc. So, if you hear any of these comments about yourself, you have precious little time to correct these impressions. Otherwise, surgery is clearly not for you.

A.   JUNIOR RESIDENT

There is a steep jump from being a medical student to becoming a resident. Suddenly, there is far more responsibility than ever before. You are now called upon to make diagnoses, initiate tests, and make decisions needed in the day-to-day management of patients. This is good training because life as a surgeon is nothing but making decisions—lots of them!—every day. The reality, though, is that there is always back up for difficult decisions. No junior resident should ever feel they are alone, with only their basic medical training and wits to guide them. If you feel like this, then it is your responsibility to speak up.

At the same time that you are learning about becoming a doctor, you are also learning about being a surgeon. Although the focus of the latter appears to emphasize technical surgery, in reality, being a surgeon is far more than that. A good surgeon is one who carefully chooses the correct patient to operate on, the correct or best operation for that patient, and then does it meticulously. The hardest thing to teach, and the aspect least appreciated by the trainee, is the patient the surgeon chooses not to operate on. The ability to discern when it is best not to operate usually comes after years of practice, together with moments of self-reflection.

As a junior resident, the thrill of being in the operating room means a chance to learn how to do surgery. Often, being able to finally handle instruments overshadows less appealing instructions, such as the importance of good posture, good lighting, and good ergonomics to prevent chronic repetitive strain injuries. Despite the flexibility of youth in your joints and eyes, a poor understanding of ergonomics will lead to future strain on your neck and lumbar spine.

Two things I find challenging for junior residents are recognizing the subtle differences in the colour of different tissues, and trying to replicate the mirror image from the opposite side of the table. For the former, colour defines anatomy and pathology. Unlike Netter's drawings in anatomy texts, most of the colours in the body are shades of brown, yellow, and red. Unfortunately, the bile duct is not bright green! Discerning the differences in colour helps to identify the various layers of tissue. This appreciation takes time and coincides with more operative experience.

The frontal and mirror images can be also be challenging, especially when standing opposite the resident while teaching. This situation arises with demonstrating how to hand tie, hold instruments, etc. Unless specially ordered, all instruments are for right-handed surgeons. This feature affects the ratchet mechanism of clamps as well as scissors. One cannot cut with scissors using your left hand while holding them exactly the way you would in your right hand.

When you start life as a brand-new resident in the OR, you are expected to observe. So, you need to carefully observe the surgeon. And after each case, you should record how the surgeon did the case—from the application of the drapes, the type of incision, the choice of instruments, any specific idiosyncrasies, any technical tips, and the closure. Surgeons are creatures of habit; they do the same thing each time. If you want to impress the same surgeon the next time, do it "their way." By doing so, it will give them some degree of comfort that you were actually observing and listening to them, and they may be willing to offer more instruction or even let you do some minor parts of the case.

While the technical teaching of surgery begins in the operating room, to become a good surgeon, you first need to be a good assistant. And to be a good assistant requires anticipating what the surgeon needs at that moment, whether it is a careful suction or applying counter traction to the surgeon's traction. An outstanding assistant makes the whole operation much simpler. If the trainee thinks that the procedure they are doing is going well, it is likely they do not notice that their hands are extensions of the surgeon's hands. The aim of the assistant is to *assist* the surgeon. That means doing whatever it takes to aid them and make the case look *easy*. You can assist in a multitude of ways. You can clear blood away from the field by wiping it with gauze sponges or using suction; improve illumination by adjusting the OR lights; and have the next instrument ready, whether it is scissors, or clamps (mosquito, artery forceps, etc.). When I was a junior resident, a senior surgeon told me, "I like to see junior residents with an instrument in each hand—it doesn't matter what it is: a sponge, snap, or cautery." Idle hands mean idle minds, so look and be prepared when in the OR.

A word about suctioning. It is an art to dart in and out of the surgical field to remove blood and fluid without disturbing the surgeon's view. The key is to not place the suction in the surgeon's field of view, a concept only recognized by understanding the mirror image view. You may also notice the surgeon using the suction to aid in dissection, providing retraction as well as suctioning. But, you better hurry—they want to do the case even if the only instrument they have is the suction!

So, raise the table to waist level, position the lights over your shoulders, and keep your hands busy with the suction, cautery, clamp, or swab. Have fun!

B. MID-LEVEL RESIDENT

By the second to third year of surgery, the mid-level resident should be well on their way in adjusting their routine to accommodate the different surgeons they work with. Each surgeon has their own style, and will teach you helpful tips you can incorporate into a style of your own.

By now, the basics of surgery should be well known: how each instrument is meant to be handled, and how to plan the case. Open and endovascular case planning is completely different. For open cases, planning is done in a progressive manner from the initial incision, dissection to encircle the vessels, proximal and distal control points, setting up the anastomosis to include placement and length of the arteriotomy, and the need to do anything local such as thromboendarterectomy, the anastomosis itself (using which technique, type of suture), completion studies, and closure of the wound.

Endovascular planning requires a wireguide platform to get to the lesion of interest, and understanding the trombone model. This means knowing what devices fit into what. Here, the planning is backwards from the final device (e.g., stent), then the steps to get there. This will mean planning the various shaped catheters, guidewires, and finally, the sheath needed after initial vascular access.

Particulars of the diseases being treated, including different options, advantages, and disadvantages, should be reviewed and discussed, and conclusions made. For instance, the treatment of carotid artery disease is based on a number of key randomized trials for symptomatic and asymptomatic carotid stenosis. But which patients do the trial findings apply to? Were the differences significant, and how large were the differences? Ultimately, can the results be applied to the patients you see?

Similarly, in the operating room, residents will see variations of technique. From these observations, key questions would be: What are the results of one type of technique compared with another? What does the literature say? Will you incorporate this into your future practice? For instance, the resident could ponder the issue of carotid patching—is it beneficial? Is there a superior material to use for patching? What would you do in the future?

For mid-level residents, surgeons want to see continual progress beyond their early years. Some residents will develop faster both in decision-making and technical ability, and these residents should be given more challenging problems. The danger in the mid-level years is when a resident reaches a plateau or regresses. Residents may need to actively seek feedback from surgeons, especially if it is not forthcoming. Deficiencies and, if necessary, attitudes need to be corrected at this stage if the resident is demonstrating poor progress. More practise, both decision-making and technical, is vital at this stage for the struggling resident.

c. SENIOR RESIDENT

By the time the resident enters their final year, they should demonstrate they are competent to practise independently. This is best exemplified by confidence in their decision-making abilities and in the operating room. They should see patients independently and express their opinion about whether an operation is required, at what time interval, and how the operation should be done. Many marginal senior residents struggle with this after years of deferring the decision-making to the attending surgeon.

In the operating room, senior residents should be given more opportunities to operate independently or with junior house staff they can teach. In the most complicated cases, surgeons want to see how the senior residents handle difficult situations and unexpected findings. They want to hear how the senior resident articulates their concern, their recommendations, and at what point they would make a recommendation for a change when the case is not proceeding smoothly. In vascular surgery, as elsewhere in life, *"Insanity is doing the same thing over and over again and expecting different results" – Albert Einstein.*

3. How to do Research as a Resident

Why do we do research? Is it because we think having publications on our resume makes it easier to get a future position? Is it for the accolades? Or is it because we may be contributing, in however small a way, to the body of knowledge called Medicine?

I remember doing my first research paper. I had no idea what we were doing and how we were going to get the data. And, finally, when we had data and somehow it got accepted for presentation, I was bombarded with questions I never thought about. Somehow, undeterred, I struggled and finished the paper, which miraculously got published (Hsiang and Hildebrand 1989).

My first experience is sadly typical of most medical students and residents who are first exposed to research. It is criminal to expect a young student or resident to spend their off hours getting data from hospital records, compiling the results, only to discover at the very end that the research is not interesting or has been previously published. So, from the resident's perspective how do you go about doing research?

The best type of research is something exciting and enthralling to do. You couldn't imagine doing anything else in your spare time but pursue that research. These examples are very uncommon, but they are admired by everybody once completed or commercialized. In vascular surgery, two successful examples are the development of the Fogarty balloon catheter by Dr. Thomas Fogarty (Fogarty et al. 1963), and the sternal saw by Dr. Ted Diethrich (Diethrich and

Morris 1963). Both innovations occurred when the inventors were medical students or junior residents.

A.   FINDING A SUPERVISOR

This is usually a neglected but, in fact, very important consideration. As the resident, you may ask a surgeon to be your mentor if you enjoy working with them. At other times, a surgeon may approach you to do research with them. However, these scenarios may or may not be successful. To do research as a resident, you need to understand your end goal. Is it to present? Publish your findings? Add to your resume? It definitely should be all of these. And unless you have some certainty that will happen, I would recommend changing something—perhaps the supervisor, the topic, etc., before you get too involved. From the mentor's perspective, are they doing this because they have an innate curiosity about a certain topic, or are they doing this to review their results for essentially an internal audit? Do they have the resident's welfare in mind when asking them to do this research?

All of the above comments are to emphasize the importance of choosing the supervisor. The right supervisor is somebody who is dedicated to the pursuit of the question and has experience in completing research to the point of publication. This frequently is the first mistake that a resident has with research—not finding the right supervisor. Apart from having a track record of successful publications, the right person to be a supervisor should hold regular research meetings to discuss progress, handle roadblocks (there will be plenty of these), get after the resident to meet key deadlines, perfect the presentation(s) with the resident, recommend appropriate journals for publication, and efficiently edit draft manuscripts.

Of all these requirements, it is the frequent meetings with the resident that is most important, since only with regular meetings are problems fleshed out and solutions developed.

B. Defining the Question

The second difficulty is defining the research question. It sounds simple, but it is not. The research question has to be all things to all people: it needs to be interesting, which usually means it is controversial; not been done before or been previously poorly described; make biologic sense; and be framed to make it a testable hypothesis. Sometimes, the proposed research is hypothesis-generating.

During this time, an early question may need to be refined according to what the previous literature has said about the topic. Do not start collecting data until the research question has been determined! Too often, residents have a vague idea, start collecting reams of data and when nothing pans out, change the research question according to the data collected. This leads to woolly thinking and lots of data that doesn't make sense. Reviewers can spot this easily and rejections will follow.

With a clear research question that can be developed into a testable hypothesis, a research design can be selected to evaluate the question. The sample population can be explicitly described, cases and controls defined, potential biases avoided, and appropriate statistical tests determined based on the available data. It is a good idea to involve a statistician early in the planning process to review the research question and chosen methodology.

C. OBTAINING ETHICS APPROVAL

Invariably, you will need ethics approval for human studies, research on animals, and handling biohazards. The ethics approval can take up to six weeks, so you need to apply for it early. They will want to know your research question and your methods. There is nothing magical about the application. Expect it to require revisions, and you should correct it according to their recommendations. If you are unsure about anything, call them and ask for clarification before sending your plan back, expecting them to understand how you interpreted their recommendations. Since ethics approval is time-limited, always ask for a longer period of study than you think you might need; otherwise, you will need to submit extensions later on.

D. WRITING AN ABSTRACT

Ideally, you will be working toward a deadline for abstract submissions. Generally, abstracts are a one-page summary of your proposal containing the Purpose or Hypothesis, Methods, Results, and Conclusion. Writing an abstract depends on what the requirements are. Most will require a blind version—meaning no author or institution names—and possibly an unblinded version. Some abstracts accept tables and figures; others don't. You can wait until the final minute to send the abstract, but if you are sure that the version you have completed is the final version, submit it. Can you imagine how frustratingly tragic it would be if a last-minute electronic glitch blocked your ability to send the abstract?

E. HOW TO WRITE AN ARTICLE

At some point, either after the abstract has been accepted or to finalize the research, your findings need to be published. All of your hard work needs a final resting place. Unfortunately, this is often the time when residents lose interest. Call it research-fatigue, or they simply have better things to do. Unpublished research represent unknown findings, and is as if you never did the work.

For maximal efficiency, the best time to start writing the paper is at the beginning, when you have finalized your research question. The format of a paper usually follows the same headings as an abstract: Background leading to the Hypothesis, Methods, Results, Discussion, and References.

The Background should include the rationale and any controversies used to develop the research question. Readers want to follow your train of thought as to why you thought the research was timely and important. The Methods section should describe the exact methods used, including sampling, definitions of cases, controls, outcomes, and statistical tests.

For the Results section, once the data has been collected and analyzed, it should be collated and displayed as tables or figures containing the relevant data from the characteristics of the study population, comparisons between cases and controls, pertinent findings, and the statistical test results. The list of References can also be started early, with the background literature.

The last remaining section will be the Discussion. Here the findings should be compared to what has been previously described in the literature. If your findings are different, then an explanation will be required describing the strengths or limitations of other authors' findings compared with yours.

If your research gets accepted as a meeting presentation, then pay close attention to questions that arise from the discussion afterwards. Incorporate any probing questions into the Discussion section in your paper as, occasionally, the very same people who asked the question may also be asked to review your paper. The key takeaway for publishing is that to get it published, prepare early, and submit the paper as soon as it is complete—when the data is the "freshest."

F.   WHERE TO PUBLISH

During the time you are writing the paper, consider where it should be published. There are many journals to choose from. Generally, aim high and choose a journal with high impact. In vascular surgery, the top-rated journal is the *Journal of Vascular Surgery*, followed by the *European Journal of Vascular Surgery*, the *Journal of Endovascular Therapy*, and *Annals of Vascular Surgery*. In addition, other surgical journals may consider vascular papers, and even medical journals may be considered, especially if your research appeals to a wider audience. Although the rejection rate from high impact journals is also higher, the reviews are far better and turnaround time is quicker than for lower impact journals (the reviewers are being reviewed as well!). Even if the paper is rejected, you may incorporate the reviewers' comments for your next submission. In short, it is unusual for manuscripts to be accepted as-is. Expect criticism and rejections from reviewers, but do not be deterred.

4. The Surgeon as Small Businessperson

One of the realities of finishing residency is that you will need to practice, not only as a surgeon, but also as a small businessperson. The "business" side of Medicine is usually not covered thoroughly, if at all, during medical school or residency. To fill this void, a number of books and seminars discussing being a physician and small businessperson are widely available (Curran 1996; Curran 2000). I will not reiterate their recommendations, but I do want to emphasize the following questions:

A.   HOW DO YOU FIND A JOB AS A SURGEON?

Some residents start thinking about this earlier, but by the time you are in your fourth or final year of residency, this question will become all-consuming. And, if you think there is a position, what constitutes a good job? And finally, how do you get that job? There may be many potential sources for job leads—your program director, who should know what positions are available in surrounding surgical practices; device manufacturers, with tips about upcoming positions; and other leads discovered by sleuthing on your own. However, the most important aspect of finding a job is that you need to *network* to let people know you are in the market. Once you have identified a job opening, is it a good job? This depends on the type of work the position offers, the location of the practice, the potential partners, and the compensation. For each possible job, you will need to decide what is acceptable and what may be a deal breaker, as finding a job that offers excellent conditions in all areas is unlikely. So, to get the job of your dreams, you need to do "recon." This includes doing an elective there. Understand the location, hospital, and surgeons. And, if needed, ask for an introduction. Above all else, have confidence when you're doing this!

B.   CAN YOU NEGOTIATE?

Once you have identified a suitable landing spot, how do you negotiate? What do you offer? What do they offer? Frequently, the young surgeon will feel so ingratiated that somebody has offered them a position that they may shortchange themselves and accept whatever the practice is offering. Most likely, the practice is looking for "new blood," but this typically means somebody to take call. If the new surgeon has additional skills, such as advanced endovascular training, that is a bonus, but the primary requirement is that they be competent and can take call without needing to call in the senior surgeons. In return, they should be willing to share their hospital resources with you. If the new position is available because a senior partner is leaving, then they need the new surgeon to join their practice to share office expenses. *Those two items, sharing call and sharing office expenses, represent 90 percent of the reasons why a practice is looking for a new surgeon.* The remaining 10 percent may be to use the new surgeon as a potential bargaining chip in the expansion of their practice, either in the OR or in the community. As a young surgeon, you may think that you have nothing to offer to a bunch of seasoned surgeons. Nothing could be further from the truth. What you have—youth, energy, ideas, and far more current knowledge, are all things they don't have! So, remember this when negotiating with your potential new partners.

C.   PARTNERS AND OFFICE EXPENSES.

When you start your career as a surgeon, nothing can be more exciting than finally operating on your own patients. However, sometimes it can be frightening since now you need to make all the decisions. Having trained so long to be a surgeon, you may feel that the OR is your natural environment. Over time though, with disrespectful behaviour aimed at surgeons from people cancelling cases, creating time delays, or bringing in new rules to control behaviour (see "Time Out"), you may realize that it is your office, and not the

OR, that is a sanctuary. In your office, at least you know when you are going to start and finish your day.

Having partners or associates can be both beneficial and a hindrance. It is definitely beneficial to start in a group practice. You can bounce ideas off your partners about difficult cases. However, you will need to know the legal obligations when a partner leaves from sickness or death, the liabilities if creditors come after a partner, and how office expenses are shared. Later in your career, you may wish to practice solo, since all the decisions, from staff to equipment, need only one person's opinion: yours.

D. DON'T BECOME DEPENDENT ON PEOPLE.

As a businessperson, you will rely on your staff to make your office more efficient, eliminate mistakes, generate better relations with patients and referring physicians, and thereby build your business. However, in the electronic era of office management, make sure that *you* can do every aspect of what your medical office assistant does. This includes everything from OR booking, transcription, data entry into the EMR, and billing.

i. Billing

Most surgeons do not do their own billing, which I find surprising. This is the most fundamental part of running your office—looking after your income. Your MOA was not in the OR at two o'clock in the morning, so how can they know what was done and how that should be billed? Learn how to bill during residency. This has the added benefit of easily recording the operations on a spreadsheet while learning how to bill. Ask about challenging billing examples and key terms to describe what was done (if there is a discrepancy between what you bill and what the billing agency is willing to pay, there will always be arbitration). I know of a horror story involving a surgeon who relied on his MOA to do all his billing, only to discover months later that she got busy with other things and did *no* billing for over six months!

ii. Staff changes

At some point, it is highly likely you will have a staff change. This could be due to illness or worse, termination. If your staff member became ill, could you do their job? Would you be able to train the replacement? That is why it is absolutely essential that you can do every aspect of their job. Similarly, have an updated job description available at all times in case you need to replace staff.

iii. Staff morale

Most of the problems in the office are interpersonal. Your staff need to understand what your preferences are, but equally, you need to provide them with encouragement and feedback about how they are doing. An annual performance review with appropriate rewards, either in terms of bonuses or paid time off, is important to let them know you appreciate their work. At the same time, you can inform them of areas where their work was excellent or could be improved. The flipside is that occasionally staff need be terminated. Prior to doing that, you should be documenting where their work is deficient, reviewing the employment standards, and possibly discussing the legal ramifications of terminating an employee with a labour lawyer.

E.   OWN YOUR OFFICE

If you plan to practice for many years in the same community, consider owning your office. It is amazing to me that most physicians do not own their office, nor ever consider it. As a renter, having a landlord responsible for fixing issues when they arise, such as plumbing problems etc., is convenient. Nonetheless, landlords may not be responsive to your needs when the hot water tank explodes, or the sinks won't drain. Your agreement to not "trash" the office and to pay rent on time is your bond with the landlord. However, rent will *always* go up. If there is an additional expense from increased property taxes to building upgrades, the cost will always be passed onto the renter. Plus, after many years of paying rent, there is no equity in your office. This is the exact opposite of owning your office. The latter means that, not only do you have complete "rent control," you also have the option of renting out part or all of your office, and years later, as most real estate would have appreciated, there is the bonus of selling your office for a capital gain. For all of these reasons, consider buying your office building or unit.

Named Manoeuvres

1. Litherland's Law: "Underneath a skin bridge will be a venous tributary"

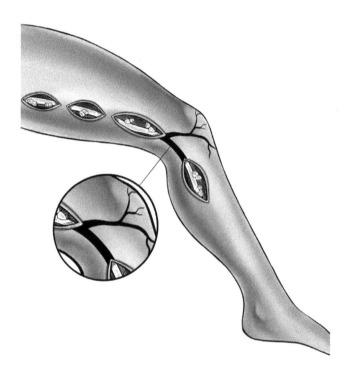

While dissecting out the great saphenous vein using multiple skin incisions, a residual side branch off the saphenous vein will often be found underneath the skin bridge. It may be the last anchoring branch when dissecting out the saphenous vein, or if an *in situ* vein bypass is performed, becomes a late arteriovenous fistula.

2. Hildebrand Hitch

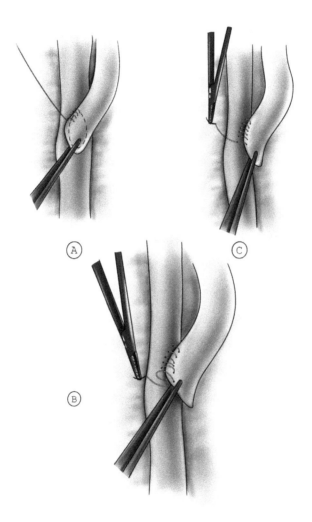

(A) When performing an anastomosis between a graft and a vessel, if one side is longer than the other, (B) take two bites on the longer side to "hitch" (shorten) it together, (C) thus making the lengths more equal.

3. Dancing on the Graft (a Peter Fry technique)

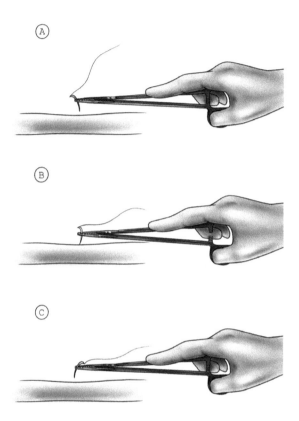

In order to have more control of the needle tip, the needle driver should grasp the curved suture needle halfway along its length and have the needle positioned 45° away from the operator. (A) If the needle ends up in an unfavourable position, the correct position can be achieved by manually adjusting the needle and needle driver by hand or by using forceps. (B) For efficiency, however, it can also be done by balancing the tip of the needle on a surface such as the bypass graft, and relax the needle driver to precisely where it needs to clasp the needle. (C) By doing so, the operator has efficiently positioned the needle on the needle driver.

4. Hsiang Technique (term coined by Gerrit Winkelaar)

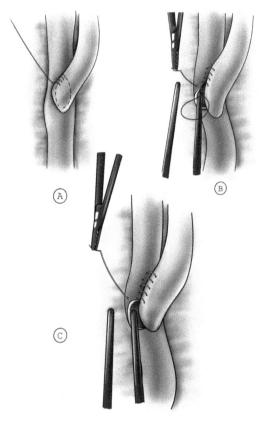

A variation of the Hildebrand Hitch, (A) when encountering a discrepancy in length between a graft and vessel, (B) gently stretch the shorter side with a blade of the forceps without grasping the vessel as you pull the suture through. This will stretch the elastic fibres in that tissue to increase its length. (C) Continue doing this until the two lengths match. (However, when anastomosing prosthetic to prosthetic material such as PTFE, where there are no elastic fibres, this should not be done as the anastomosis will then be too tight).

5. Laying the Suture Flat (a Hsiang technique)

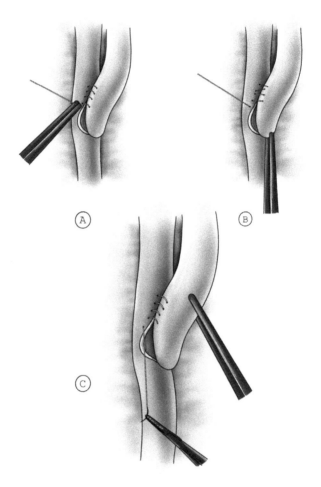

To keep sutures spaced neatly when anastomosing, various techniques including (A) using open forceps to guide the suture can be used. However, when suturing without an assistant, (B) holding the graft while pulling the suture through often leads to the suture lying in an uneven fashion. (C) This can be overcome by pulling the suture in the direction of the distal artery rather than at right angles to the anastomosis.

6. The Releasing Tie (a Hsiang technique)

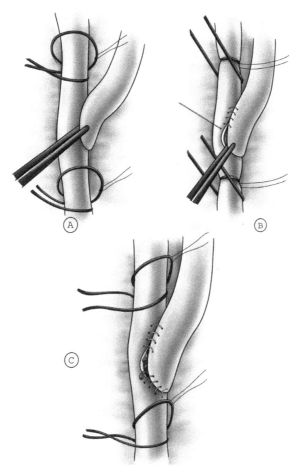

When operating on small vessels, for hemostatic control, (A) vessels can be double-looped with small vessel loops. (B) In order to facilitate prompt vessel loop release, a second suture is passed through the double loop and this serves as the releasing tie. (C) To restore blood flow, the releasing tie is pulled first, thereby loosening the double loop. This is a simple and efficient method to restore flow without the use of microclamps.

References

1. Luxton, Donald. 2006. *Vancouver General Hospital: 100 Years of Care and Service*. Vancouver: Vancouver Coastal Health.

2. Dente C. J., Feliciano D. V. 2005 "Alexis Carrel (1873-1944)." *Archives of Surgery* 140:609-10.

3. DeBakey M. E., Simeone F. A. 1946. "Battle injuries of the arteries in World War II; An analysis of 2,471 cases." *Annals of Surgery* 123:534-79.

4. Couch N. P. 1989. "About heparin, or…Whatever happened to Jay MacLean?" *Journal of Vascular Surgery* 10:1-8.

5. Hess H. 1992. "Obituary: Jean Kunlin." *European Journal of Vascular Surgery* 6:442-43.

6. Smith R. B. 1993. "Arthur B. Voorhees, Jr.: Pioneer vascular surgeon." *Journal of Vascular Surgery* 18:341-48.

7. Dubost C., Allary M., Oeconomos N. 1951. "Treatment of aortic aneurysms; removal of the aneurysm; re-establishment of continuity by grafts of human aorta." *Mémoires Académie Chirurgie (Paris)* 77:381-83.

8. Bergqvist D. 2008. "Historical aspects of aneurysmal disease." *Scandinavian Journal of Surgery* 97:90-99.

9. Friedman S. G. 2014. "The first carotid endarterectomy." *Journal of Vascular Surgery* 60:1703-8.

10. Yao J. S. T. 2010. "Society for Vascular Surgery (SVS)–The Beginning." *Journal of Vascular Surgery* 51:776-9.

11. Patterson, Frank P. 2000. *The Cutting Edge.* Hatzic Publishing.

12. Chung W. B. 1979. "The carotid body tumour." *Canadian Journal of Surgery* 22:319.

13. Chen J. C., Salvian A. J., Taylor D. C., Teal P. A., Marotta T. R., Hsiang Y. N. 1998. "Predictive ability of duplex ultrasonography for internal carotid artery stenosis of 70 to 99 percent: a comparative study." *Annals of Vascular Surgery* 12:244-247.

14. Chen J. C., Hildebrand H. D., Salvian A. J., Taylor D. C., Hsiang Y. N. 1996. "Predictors of mortality in non-ruptured and ruptured abdominal aortic aneurysms." *Journal of Vascular Surgery* 24:614-623.

15. Chen J. C., Hsiang Y. N., Morris C. M., Benny W. B. 1996. "Cocaine-induced multiple vascular occlusions: A case report." *Journal of Vascular Surgery* 23(4):719-723.

16. Hsiang Y. N., Crespo M. T., Todd M. E. 1995. "Dosage and timing of Photofrin for photodynamic therapy of intimal hyperplasia." *Cardiovascular Surgery* 3:489-494.

17. Curtis S. B., Hewitt J., Yakubovitz S., Anzarut A., Hsiang Y. N., Buchan A. M. 2000. "Somatostatin receptor subtype expression in human vascular tissue." *American Journal of Physiology.* Heart Circ Physiology 278 (6), pp. H 1815-1822.

18. Thompson J. E. 1997. "Carotid surgery–the past is prologue." *Journal of Vascular Surgery* 25:131-40.

19. Chung W. B. 1967. "Carotid artery surgery for cerebrovascular insufficiency." *Canadian Journal of Surgery* 10:21-27.

20. Brent, L. 1997. *A history of transplantation immunology.* Academic Press.

21. Harvard Gazette. 2011. *A transplant makes history.* Sept. 22, 2001.

22. Siegel B. 1998. "A Brief History of Doppler Ultrasound in the diagnosis of Peripheral Vascular disease." *Ultrasound Medical Biology* 24:169-176.

23. Gupta K. N., Palmer M., Cheeseman C. 2003. "Comparison of medical students' elective choices before and after abolition of rotating internships." *Medical Education* 37:470-1.

24. Glauser W. 2018. "Canada's medical residency system is leaving some graduates in limbo." *University Affairs.* Apr 4, 2018.

25. Friedman S.G. 1989. "Charles Dotter: interventional radiologist." *Radiology* 172:921-24.

26. UC Davis Health. 2010. *Julio Palmaz: Inventor of the first commercially available stent.* Fall 2010.

27. Hsiang Y. N., Todd M. E., Crespo M. T., Machan L. S. 1994. "Intraluminal endothelium-covered bridges in chronic fat-fed balloon-injured Yucatan miniswine." *Journal of Investigative Surgery* 7(6):541-50.

28. Hsiang Y. N., Houston G. T. M., Crespo M. T., To E., Sobeh M. S., Todd M. E., Bower R. D. 1995. "Preventing intimal hyperplasia with photodynamic therapy using an intravascular probe." *Annals of Vascular Surgery* 9:80-86.

29. Schajer G. S., Green S. I., Davis A. P., Hsiang Y. N. 1996. "Influence of elastic non-linearity on arterial anastomotic compliance." *Journal of Mechanical Engineering* 118:445-451.

30. Canadian Institute for Health Information 2007. *HSMR: A new approach for measuring hospital mortality trends in Canada.*

31. Barer M. L., Stoddart G. L. 1992. "Toward integrated Medical resource policies for Canada: 1. Background, process and perceived problems." *Canadian Medical Association Journal* 146:347-351.

32. Barer M. L., Stoddart G. L. 1992. "Toward integrated Medical resource policies for Canada: 2. Promoting change—general themes." *Canadian Medical Association Journal* 146:697-700.

33. Evans R. G., McGrail K. M. 2008. "Richard III, Barer-Stoddart and the daughter of time." *Healthcare Policy* 3(3) 18-28 doi:10.12927/hcpol.2008.19564.

34. Esmail N. 2016. "Canada's physician supply." *Canadian Student Review*. Winter 2016:33-41.

35. Patrick A. B. 2000. "Putting together pieces of the physician supply puzzle." *Canadian Medical Association Journal* 162:313-314.

36. Stoddart G. L., Barer M. L. 1999. "Will increasing medical school enrolment solve Canada's physician supply problems?" *Canadian Medical Association Journal* 161:983-984.

37. Barer M. L., Stoddart G. L. 1991. "Toward integrated medical resource policies for Canada." Report prepared for the Federal/Provincial/Territorial Conference of Deputy Ministers of Health, June 1991.

38. *Closer to Home*: "The Report of the British Columbia Royal Commission on Health Care and Costs." 1991.

39. Litherland H. K. 1993. *Vascular Surgery 2001. Report of the COUTH/UBC Division of Vascular Surgery Strategic Planning Committee.* April 23, 1993.

40. Hickman R. O., Buckner C. D., Clift R. A., Sanders J. E., Stewart P., Thomas E. D. 1979. "A modified right atrial catheter for access to the venous system in marrow transplant recipients." *Surgery Gynecology Obstet*rics. 148 (6):871–5.

41. Broviac J. W., Cole J. J., Scribner B. H. 1973. "A silicone rubber atrial catheter for prolonged parenteral alimentation." *Surgery Gynecology Obstetrics* 136 (4):602–6.

42. Parodi J. C., Palmaz J. C., Barone H. D. 1991. "Transfemoral intraluminal graft implantation for abdominal aortic aneurysms." *Annals of Vascular Surgery* 5:491-9.

43. Flood C. M., Sullivan T. 2005. "Supreme disagreement: The highest court affirms an empty right." *Canadian Medical Association Journal.* 173:142 -43.

44. Editorial. 2005. *Canadian Medical Association Journal.* 173:117.

45. Simpson J. 2014. "The health accord was a "fix" we must not repeat." *Globe and Mail.* Apr 2, 2014.

46. Eliminating Code Gridlock in Canada's Health Care System. 2015. Wait Time Alliance Report Card. pp. 1-15.

47. North American Symptomatic Carotid Endarterectomy Trial Collaborators (NASCET). 1991. "Beneficial effect of carotid endarterectomy in symptomatic patients with high-grade stenosis." *New England Journal of Medicine* 325:445-53.

48. European Carotid Surgery Trialists' (ECST) Collaborative Group. 1991. "MRC European carotid surgery trial: interim

results with severe (70-99%) or with mild (0-29%) carotid stenosis." *Lancet* 337:1235-43.

49. Turnbull R. G., Taylor D. C., Hsiang Y. N., Salvian A. J., Nanji S., O'Hanley G., Doyle D. L., Fry P. D. 2000. "Assessment of patient waiting times for vascular surgery." *Canadian Journal of Surgery* 43:105-111.

50. Eggerton L. 2005. "Wait Time Alliance first to set benchmarks." *Canadian Medical Association Journal* 172:1277.

51. Haynes A. B., Weiser T. G., Berry W. R., et al. 2009. A surgical safety checklist to reduce morbidity and mortality in a global population." *New England Journal of Medicine* 360:191-99.

52. Urbach D. R., Govindarajan A., Saskin R., Wilton A. S., Baxter N. N. 2014. "Introduction of surgical safety checklists in Ontario, Canada." *New England Journal of Medicine* 370; 11:1029-1038.

53. Chen X., Assadasangabi B., Hsiang Y. N., Takahata K. 2018. "Enabling angioplasty-ready "smart" stents to detect in-stent restenosis and occlusion." *Advanced Science.* 2018 10.1002/advs.201700560.

54. Yi Y., Chen J., Hsiang Y. N., Takahata K. 2019. "Wirelessly heating stents via radiofrequency resonance toward enabling endovascular hyperthermia." *Advances in Healthcare Materials*, 2019 doi:10.1002/adhm.201900708.

55. Litherland, Henry K. *Memoirs of a Lancashire Lad*. (Unpublished).

56. Hildebrand, Hilda K. 2006. *Reflections*. Rosetta Projects.

57. Hildebrand, Henry D. 2006. *Tides and Times: A life story*. Rosetta Projects.

58. Hsiang Y. N. 2020. "Presidential Address: An ode to waves and trainees." *Journal of Vascular Surgery.* 71:1075-6.

59. Obituary 2008: Henry Hildebrand. *Canadian Medical Association Journal,* 2008; 178:1511.

60. Fry P. D. 1991. "Presidential Address, 1989. The future of Vascular Surgery in Canada." *Canadian Jfournal of Surgery* 34:231-236.

61. Lokanathan R., Palerme L., Salvian A. J., Taylor D. C., Hsiang Y. N. 2001. "Outcome after thrombolysis and selective thoracic outlet decompression for primary axillary vein thrombosis." *Journal of Vascular Surgery* 33:783-8.

62. Moneta G. L., Taylor D. C., Helton W. S., Mulholland M. W., Strandness D. E. 1988. "Duplex ultrasound measurement of post-prandial intestinal blood flow: effect of meal composition." *Gastroenterology* 95:1294-1301.

63. Baxter K. A., Laher I., Church J., Hsiang Y. N. 2006. "Acidosis augments myogenic constriction in rat coronary arteries." *Annals of Vascular Surgery* 20:630-7.

64. Misskey J. D., Yang C., MacDonald S., Hsiang Y. N. 2015. "A comparison of RUDI and DRIL for the management of severe access-related hand ischemia." *Journal of Vascular Surgery* 62:535-536.

65. Misskey J., Hamidazadeh R., Chen J. C., Faulds J. M., Gagnon J., Hsiang Y. N. 2020. "Influence of arterial and venous diameters on autogenous arteriovenous access patency." *Journal of Vascular Surgery* 71:158-72.

66. Vascular Access: 2018 Clinical Practice Guidelines of the European Society for Vascular Surgery (ESVS).

European Journal of Vascular and Endovascular Surgery doi:10.1016/j.ejvs.2018.02.001.

67. Huber T. 2020. "Optimizing arteriovenous fistula patency." *Journal of Vascular Surgery* 71:173.

68. Grenon S. M., Gagnon J., Hsiang Y. N. 2009. "Ankle-Brachial Index for Assessment of Peripheral Arterial Disease." *New England Journal of Medicine* 361:e40.

69. Hsiang Y. N., Hildebrand H. D. 1989. "Results of vascular surgery in younger versus older patients." *American Journal of Surgery* 157:419422.

70. Fogarty T. J., Cranley J. J., Krause R. J., Strasser E. S., Hafener C. D. 1963. "A method for extraction of arterial emboli and thrombi." *Surgery Gynecology & Obstetrics* 116: 241.

71. Diethrich E. B., Morris J. D. 1963. "Sternal saw—new instrument for splitting the sternum." *Surgery* 53:637-8.

72. Curran, Terry. 1996. *Prescription for Wealth: Financial planning for the health care professional.* Crowne Rock.

73. Curran, Terry. 2000. *Second Opinion. Hire the best financial advisor or do it yourself.* Crowne Rock.

Acronyms Used

AAA	abdominal aortic aneurysm
AKA	above knee amputation
AVF	arteriovenous fistula
ATLS	Advanced Trauma Life Support
ATS	American Transplant Society
CDMH	Conference of Deputy Ministers of Health
CEA	carotid endarterectomy
CIHI	Canada Institute for Health Information
COUTH	Council for University Teaching Hospitals
CSVS	Canadian Society for Vascular Surgery
ECG	electrocardiogram
EMR	electronic medical records
ENT	Ear, Nose, and Throat
ER	emergency room
EVAR	endovascular aneurysm repair
FUFA	fucked up femoral artery
HKU	Hong Kong University
HSMR	hospital standardized mortality ratio
ICU	intensive care unit
LOS	length of stay
MRSA	methicillin resistant *Staphyloccocus aureus*

MOA	medical office assistant
NASCET	North American Symptomatic Carotid Endarterectomy Trial
NHS	National Health Service (UK)
OR	operating room
PI	principal investigator
PPE	personal protective equipment
PTFE	polytetrafluoroethylene
R4	fourth year resident
RA	Royal Air Force (UK)
RN	registered nurse
SPH	St. Paul's Hospital
SVS	Society for Vascular Surgery
UBCH	University of British Columbia Hospital
UCSF	University of California San Francisco
VA	Veteran's Affairs
VGH	Vancouver General Hospital